ALOPECIA, IT'S A THING!
BREAKING THROUGH THE
B.S. (BELIEF SYSTEMS)

How to Overcome the Emotional Struggles
Associated With Hair Loss

Stephanie Anderson, DPC, MPC, BSM

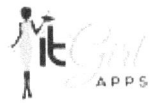

IT Girl Apps Publications

For more information, or to book an event, contact :

alopeciaitsathing@gmail.com

www.alopeciaitsathing.com

Editing by Marcel A. Anderson Jr.

ISBN: 979-8-218-14226-1 (Paperback)

Dedicated to those of you who are wondering if you can benefit from anything in this book. Yes, you CAN!

Marcel A. Anderson, Jr. (Bush), my husband. You are more than my "better half", you are my "best complete". Our wonderful sons, Vonray, Christian (Nikke), and Tristan; our grandchildren Beaux and Hosea O.M. To my parents, Hosea and Bertha Robinson.

My sister and BFF, Jesslyn, and brother Hosea B. To all of you who are living with Alopecia, you are the inspiration for this book.

CONTENTS

FOREWORD
Rodney Barnett and Carolyn Stovall

Rodney Barnett

I met Stephanie Anderson over 10 years ago when I was looking for a professional in her area of expertise, non-surgical hair replacement (NSHR). There was a void in my hair loss services—a need for non-surgical hair replacement, for which I consider her one of the foremost authorities on the subject.

She quickly filled that void and made her extensive knowledge of hair loss available to many of my colleagues, whom I had trained over the years. Because of her unselfishness and willingness to share her knowledge, we formed a partnership and came up with a way to teach, train, and certify people who want to work in the multibillion-dollar hair loss industry.

She has created a series of DVDs (some of which we've created together) on hair loss, so it was not a surprise when she shared her desire to write a book with me. Though she realized that there have been several books written on the subject of hair loss, she approaches the subject from a unique standpoint.

Rodney Barnett, Certified Trichologist and Natural Health Professional

Carolyn Stovall

1 Corinthians 11:15 "But if a woman have long hair, it is a glory to her: for her hair is given for a covering."

Hair is a covering, having a covering means a veil. The long hair of a woman is her veil. In The Bible, long hair distinguishes a man from a woman. Hair represents health and beauty in youth, wisdom, and vitality in old age as the color turns to grey. Some say that the outward appearance of our hair reflects the inner glory of God's character being developed within us. The Amish believe that The Bible instructs women to let their hair grow to rise above secular fashion. In some evangelical Christians, long hair is used as a sign of humility.

So, the question is what is "glory"? The Hebrew word is Kavod; this has meant "importance", "weight", "deference", "heaviness", "respect", "glory", "honor", and "majesty".

We know that hair has been considered one of the important and prominent aspects of our physical appearance. It is the first thing we notice when we see someone. In all nations and all cultures, people give a lot of attention to their own hair and the hair of others. My mother is 92 years old and still loves her hair; she feels it is her crown and glory. It makes her feel good to have it maintained. It also worries her that her hair is thinning out and that she has bald spots.

As an African American, I can say that we as women longed for, and envied those with long hair. As you look around today, many women have incorporated different types of weaves in their hair, or wigs, to achieve the satisfaction of long hair.

However, in the 1900s, long hair changed, and women began to cut their hair into what we call "bobs". This hairstyle was considered scandalous in those days. Hollywood movies ushered in the trend for short hair and now is a very acceptable fashion statement. Through Vogue magazine (1892), Mademoiselle (1935), and Glamour (1935), women were introduced to hairstyle and fashion. Today it does not matter what kind of hairstyle you wear.

But what about the woman who has lost her hair? How does that affect her image of herself? In 1 Peter 3:3-4, the scriptures read, "Whose adorning let it not be that outward adorning of plaiting the hair, and of wearing of gold, or of putting on apparel; But let it be the hidden man of the heart, in that which is not corruptible, even the ornament of a meek and quiet spirit, which is in the sight of God of great price."

I am a woman who had a lot of hair, thick hair. I did not like my hair and often thought of cutting it off. I hated the upkeep of my hair and sitting long hours at a beauty shop. Most of the time I did it myself. I could appreciate the long hair of others but did not want it for myself. I believe that long hair opened different opportunities for black women. It identified closer to the white woman. As children, we loved playing with white dolls with long hair. Mattel got smart and made more money when they made black dolls with long hair.

I am a Cancer survivor and have undergone Chemotherapy where I lost all of my hair. When it started falling out, I felt empowered when I made the decision to shave my head. I chose not to wear a head wrap or hat, but to sport baldness—my new identity. I remember when Grace Jones sported her baldness; she was beautiful. I was beautiful. Today my hair has grown back, the texture has changed again. I do not like my hair or the maintenance of my hair. Others think it is gorgeous and soft. I wear it proudly for those who cannot, for some reason, grow their hair.

I am reminded that in Matthew 10:30, the scriptures say "But the very hairs of your head are all numbered." This tells me that

God still knows how many hair follicles I have, seen or unseen. He created them...

Carolyn Stovall. B.A. in Psychology and Sociology and a minor in Women's Studies from Bellevue College (Bellevue, Nebraska). She also has a Master's in Community Counseling from St. Mary's University (San Antonio, Texas).

PREFACE

I n addition to Trichology and Hair Replacement services, I conduct a good amount of individual coaching in my line of work. Many of these people are struggling with emotional problems in their life, which frequently have hair loss as a contributing factor. When I am asked to speak to siblings, coworkers, family, and friends, who have been sent to me by people I have helped over the years, I also offer self-esteem and confidence coaching. God had other plans for my life and ministry than I ever had. Recently, it seems like He's been calling me to provide advice more frequently. This kind of labor was never in my life's plan. People who attend my international training, view my videos on various platforms, or tune in to my weekly TV program frequently approach me with inquiries, advice, and requests for prayer.

I do not aim to reveal any sensitive information in this book, and I will not mention any specific people unless I have their consent. Others, "the names have been changed to protect the innocent". The concerns I discuss may be relevant to you or someone you know, but keep in mind that I'm speaking generally about the most serious situations people approach me with, not specifically about anyone in particular.

People today are dealing with a variety of issues as they make the best of this difficult, personal, and emotional circumstance. Many people are suffering from intolerable conditions and have for a very long time; their situation has not improved.

What's the big deal with hair loss, you might be asking. Everyone eventually loses their hair, right? There is no purpose in purchasing a book on it. In any case, how much more is there to say about hair loss? And isn't worrying about hair loss pretty pointless when a global pandemic is still going on?

I would never suggest that COVID-19 and its variants should be given less attention than hair loss. I do believe that there is a lot to be said about it, particularly the B.S. (Belief Systems) that emerge as a result of it. I wrote this book for that reason. I firmly believe that losing your hair may be a devastating blow to your self-esteem and that it can have an impact on your social life, professional performance, and self-perception.

The fact of the matter is that there are steps you can do to slow down or stop hair loss as well as methods for getting a brand-new head of hair; including surgery and non-surgical hair replacement if you chose to go that path. By taking into account additional choices that will be covered later in this book, you may be able to comprehend the severity of the hair loss issue.

This book is specifically for you. Whether you have already experienced significant hair loss, or are simply observing the hair (or lack thereof) of other family members and fearing that you will soon experience hair loss, this book will help you address your worries, sort through and weigh your options in the most useful manner.

Hair loss – or Alopecia, is one of those subjects that elicit varying responses depending on who you are. If you are not affected by hair loss, it is likely that you are not concerned about it. But if you are one of the millions of people who experience hair loss, it may be on your mind every waking moment of the day. Alopecia can be temporary or permanent; this can affect just your scalp or the entirety of your body. It could be brought on by hereditary factors, hormonal changes, illnesses, or a natural aspect of aging. Anyone can experience hair loss and the many changes associated with it.

Many of those changes associated with losing your hair are appearance related and considered devastating for many. This may affect how you and other people see you. As a practicing Trichologist and Certified Hair Replacement Professional, I have worked with many clients living with hair loss. I have trained other licensed professionals on how to provide service to this special demographic of clients.

Over the years, I have had countless clients share the emotional toll losing their hair has caused them. The thought of losing their hair is unbearable, let alone actually seeing the visible results in the mirror. For many, they have refused to look at themselves without their cranial prostheses, wigs, hair toppers, hats, or other head coverings on. Others have shared battling depression, self-esteem issues, and lack of confidence due to losing their hair.

I too have encountered those clients who have come to grips with their hair loss. Although ideally, those clients preferred the days when they didn't have to worry about hair loss, they learned to accept it and others embraced it. Those who found their way to not suffer from hair loss but to live with it, I noticed most developed a higher level of self-esteem and self-confidence.

My years of experience behind the chair have given me the opportunity to work with clients on opposite ends of the spectrum. Those who have hair loss concerns and those who do not. There is a great distinction in relation to the way clients viewed themselves and hair loss has allowed me the opportunity to gain a little insight. Also, having years of experience behind the chair, prior to working in the hair loss industry, I have observed the reaction from others to those who have hair loss. There is undoubtedly a stigma associated with those living with hair loss. Whether intentionally or unintentionally, there is a demographic of people in our society who are very critical of others...even against those who have been diagnosed with Alopecia. This scrutiny, I feel, adds to the self-conscious and overwhelming feelings of insecurity felt by many losing their hair.

My initial concept for this book was to: bring awareness to hair loss, eradicate the stigma of hair loss and provide emotional support to those with Alopecia. Also, to share my journey of service to assist other professionals that seek to serve this special demographic of clients too. Whew, chile...that's a lot to cover in one book!

Early in my writing process, I came to the reality of the proverbial saying, "Rome wasn't built in a day", which is true. Meaning, it takes time and effort to complete a difficult activity or reach a large goal, and that I should not try to rush myself. Who knows how long it would take to create a body of work containing everything I'd like to cover.

As an educator, my heart and intentions are to teach and share. Attempting to thoroughly address each topic identified is going to have to be done in more than just one writing. So, I decided to address one of the most important topics that have become near and dear to my heart. Trying to provide emotional support to those with Alopecia. Hopefully, while expounding on this particular subject, some of the other important issues may come into view as well. This will be the first book headed to publishing.

As a result of events in the last few years, so much has changed. The COVID-19 pandemic has had significant and far-reaching effects on health systems, the economy, and the world. It is one of the largest global disasters in generations. Numerous people have lost their lives or their means of support. Communities and families have been torn apart and stressed. Learning and social interaction have been lost for children and teenagers.

There have been business failures. I am so eternally thankful that my business did not suffer permanent closure as a result. It has proven to be a resource for those clients seeking hair loss services as well as additional care. "What does this have to do with hair loss?", you ask. EVERYTHING!!!

Mental health has been severely impacted as people deal with these health, social, and economic effects. It has been exacerbated by those living with hair loss. People feel isolated, not socializing, working and/or studying from home, and hiding behind Zoom video conference meetings using audio only. Many of us experienced increased anxiety, but for others of us, COVID-19 may have further worsened already existing mental health issues. The symptoms of despair, anxiety, and post-traumatic stress disorder have all been widely described, as well as psychological distress. I have noticed more clients in my care expressing more concerns regarding self-esteem, anxiety, and depression. Self-care is currently a popular buzzword.

I have often wondered why so many people have low or negative self-esteem and why, despite their best efforts, they never seem to be able to achieve high self-esteem. I came to the conclusion that people are waging a losing war as long as they base their self-esteem on what other people think of them. Self-esteem is based on the daily behaviors we engage in for our own sake, not those we engage in for the sake of earning the respect of others. No matter how much we love ourselves, it will not matter if what other people think of us is what drives our self-esteem.

Until you acknowledge and reduce your other-esteeming (which I will cover later), you will ultimately struggle to value yourself regardless of hair loss. That's why I invite you to read this book on Alopecia with an open mind and strong optimism. I will share how to break through the B.S. (belief systems). Regardless of how (personally or otherwise) you are affected by hair loss.

"...But David encouraged himself in the Lord" *(1 Samuel 30:6)*.

Let's be like King David, in moments of distress we can encourage ourselves. To do this, my favorite Bible scriptures about beauty and self-worth are shared with you throughout this book. You're not the only one who has trouble with how you look when you look in the mirror. The beauty expectations of society can be brutal. But we must swap out that callous attitude for a kinder, gentler approach for ourselves. Let's look at what The Bible says about our beauty from God's perspective, rather than focusing on what the mainstream media wants us to think about inner and outer beauty.

You can believe that God, who speaks to us through the inspired words of The Bible, has the best perspective available to us. Look no further if you want to raise your self-esteem a little.

For these verses, I chose a variety of translations. To make it easier for you to locate the verse you're looking for, here is a brief key.

Name of Version	Abbreviation
American Standard Version	ASV
English Standard Version	ESV
King James Version	KJV
New International Version	NIV
New Living Version	NLV

There is more to it than just supplying you with some encouragement along this journey. Another objective of this writing is to increase your awareness of the options available to you if you are experiencing hair loss; to increase your comfort level in pursuing those options, and feel confident in your decision-making process. I want you to be an informed and secure customer whether you decide to use topicals, take medicine, purchase a hair unit (non-surgical hair replacement), or proceed directly with hair transplantation (surgical hair replacement).

Additionally, I want you to comprehend hair—what it is, why it responds the way it does to the abuse most of us dump on it, and the best ways to maintain its aesthetic quality and decimate the B.S. (Belief Systems) that hinder many.

These pages contain representations of every woman with hair loss I've known, loved, and worked with over the past two-plus decades. My capacity to aid them was influenced by their experiences. I especially consider the women who were gradually "dying" emotionally as a result of their low confidence and low self-esteem. A large number of those women triumphantly rediscovered their identities and realized their significance once more. I know, having been afforded the opportunity to help them, others and myself are standing on their shoulders.

I want you to know, you are more valuable than the many sparrows or other animals on the Earth because God loves you. Be heartened by the fact that God loves you so much if you're going through a difficult period. You are God's most exquisite and flawless creation, so try to maintain a kind and tranquil spirit. You have access to eternal life in paradise via Jesus Christ. I pray that this collection of Bible passages on beauty and worth will boost your self-confidence today.

CHAPTER 1

CLASS IS IN SESSION

Alopecia, Roll Call

Alopecia, it's a thing! Roll call for a few of those who have it: it's a thing that Monica worries about late at night. It's a thing that has robbed Kaye of her confidence. It's a thing that keeps Stacey from attending social events. It's a thing that compels Alisha to stare at strangers who have it. It's a thing that Debbie has lived with since the age of nine. It's a thing that Farah has experienced after having a baby; etc. The roll call could go on continuously, but I think you get the picture. No one with Alopecia should ever feel alone, isolated, or like they are the only one. Alopecia is an undeniable game changer and no respecter of person, age, or sex...you get it—Alopecia, it's a thing!

My ambition for this book is to educate the reader about hair loss and breaking through the B.S. that is most times associated with it. So, regardless of what you know about hair loss, I would be remiss not to provide a cursory review of the subject.

By all means, if the snippet of information I share with you drives you to a desire to learn more, then please do your due diligence and do a deep dive and educate yourself on the subject.

Not Your Ordinary

Practically speaking, class is in session. Within the covers of this book is an instrument designed to explain the fundamentals of hair loss, scalp difficulties, and other topics that are less frequently discussed. It's not your ordinary book on Alopecia. This book was created to support those who care for and support women who are experiencing hair loss, scalp maladies, and emotional problems. Whether personally or in a professional capacity.

If you work as a Hair Stylist, you surely notice that more and more of your clients are experiencing hair loss and thinning. It's okay if you're unsure of how to assist these special clients. I hope that this information will inspire you to connect with Trichologists and Hair Loss Specialists in your area. Also, to clarify why it is essential to give these clientele extra amenities. If you work as a Trichologist, Hair Loss Practitioner, Hair Replacement Specialist, or another type of Hair Loss Professional, you are aware of the value of having a wide range of resources at your disposal for your customers who are experiencing hair loss. This book is an excellent tool to help with hair loss, as well as the underlying secondary disorders linked with it if you are a Dermatologist, Oncologist, or other Medical Professional who does not specialize in hair and scalp illnesses. The book will undoubtedly be helpful to you if you're a layperson experiencing scalp or hair loss issues. After reading it, you'll know exactly where to look for assistance for both issues seen and unseen.

The moment has come to act decisively. You may look up information on hair loss for women online. The search yields a dizzying array of remedies, goods, and services. How do you decide what to believe, what is true, and what is false? Even conversations with medical professionals reveal varying viewpoints on what is beneficial and what is not. In my facility where I interact with clients every day, there has always been an underlying current related to the emotional aspect of losing one's hair. Not much is spoken about it. But as COVID-19 increased, like many aspects of our life, I started to see more instances and a need to help my clients support their mental and emotional health, along with engaging in "self-care."

What You Think and Feel

I am all here for the B.S. (Belief Systems), mindset, and biases. Yes, biases; everyone has biases, but often we don't realize them. Challenging the mindsets that tend to limit you, plus discovering why and how they possibly impact you and what can be done to manage or change them.

Is self-esteem just really a "Belief System"? YES! It undoubtedly is! What you think and ultimately feel about yourself constitutes your self-esteem; this is when you think of it as a set of beliefs. It becomes a system of belief or "Belief System" when it helps you interpret your everyday reality. What you hold true about what is or should be, what's right or wrong, what's true or false.

Many people find this hard to accept and would rather assume that self-esteem is something that one is "born" with and that one cannot develop. This is untrue, if you think back on your life, you can definitely recall instances when you felt "wonderful" and "full of confidence". For instance, passing the final exam in a major course or class was a significant moment in life. If you've ever had to audition for anything and you made the cut, didn't that make you feel "on top of the world"?

When you think about self-esteem in these terms, you'll undoubtedly realize that it has probably fluctuated a lot during your life; from periods when it was quite low to other times when you were "on cloud nine"!

So, when it comes to the sensitive, unsettling, and often devastating topic that is hair loss, many clients are experiencing plummeting self-esteem levels. Breaking through the negative B.S. with compassion, this book gives women hope and much-needed help in the struggle against this little-discussed, but very real, epidemic of hair loss and its emotional aspects. Throughout the book, you will see the words Alopecia and Hair Loss used interchangeably. In all sincerity, it's not my attempt to confuse you because typically, they have the same meaning. However, there are some specific types of Alopecia that you will benefit from distinguishing one from another.

* * *

Dear Friend, I pray that you enjoy good health and that all may go well with you, even as your soul is getting along well. *3 John 1:2 (NIV)*

CHAPTER 2

UNDERSTANDING HAIR LOSS

My Personal Journey

M ost people aren't concerned about hair loss unless it affects them or someone they care about. I can honestly say many, many, many years ago, that statement probably included me as well. Like many, it wasn't that I didn't care, I just didn't comprehend totally how losing hair can affect someone. Even as a licensed stylist, my experience and knowledge of hair loss, along with those clients losing their hair took time to nurture a deeper understanding.

Thirty years ago, as a cosmetology student, what I learned about Alopecia (hair loss) was just a page-and-a-half snippet of information in a textbook of 634 pages. Learning how to care for, maintain and style healthy hair took priority early on. It was only after many years of practicing cosmetology services in real life did I truly get introduced to hair loss and its effect on clients.

Early on in my career within cosmetology, it afforded me the opportunity to provide services by helping my clients look and feel great. Just by simply caring for, maintaining, and styling their hair, my clients would purely morph into different people by the end of their appointment. My first salon was a co-ownership called "B4 and After", because of the looks created for our clients. Cosmetology also allowed me to exhibit my creativity and assist my clients in expressing their personalities through my hair styling services.

Dream Weaver

The "sew-in" weave was the most requested service I provided in the 1990s. I worked hard to integrate the commercial hair with the client's natural hair for the most realistic look possible. The key was to ensure that the foundation (braids) was secure and the tracks were flat. Eventually, I started offering more sophisticated methods like the interlocking, braid-less, net weave, etc.; the same concept, but the execution was different. Ninety-five (95%) percent of my clients had no hair loss issues; they just wanted to have different styling options. The other small percentage that did so had only minor thinning and no extensive hair loss or Alopecia. Many of them couldn't grow hair as long as they wanted, so we utilized the hair weave to add length and density (fullness).

Of course, they wanted their hair to look as natural as possible. Of which, I obliged. So, imagine this back in the day, there was such a stigma of people wearing weaves that every six to eight weeks my client, we'll say, Ms. Smith, came in for a sew-in service. She would receive a sew-in removal and reinstallation. At each reinstallation appointment, I would add either 1/2" to 3/4" in length. Why, you asked? Good question. The natural growth rate of healthy hair is normally one-half inch (1/2") per month or six inches (6") per year. I actually had to take out my tape measure to make sure of the length. She wanted her sew-in weave to appear as if her hair were "growing" and that it was all hers and not artificial hair.

Remember, this was Oklahoma City, OK, in the '90s; decades before it became fashionable to wear wigs, weaves, and extensions. This was the time in which it was a mark of disgrace for many of my clients to think others knew they were wearing anything but their own hair. I didn't understand it then...the psychological impact that was being exhibited here.

The lengths that Ms. Smith and others were willing to go to in order for their "secret" to not be revealed. Now, that held true for many of my clients, but there were a handful of others that had no inhibitions when it came to wearing artificial hair. They changed it up every chance they got. They went from the extreme of lengths, colors, textures, etc., without a care in the world of who thought what. Their only concern was whether or not they looked "fly" in it. Yep, looking "fly" was a good thing back then. It wasn't a put down...not at all. Yet, again...I didn't realize the significance of the opposing views I was observing when it came to clients. It took some time for me to come to that "A-ha" moment about the psychology of it all; and when I mean, some time, I mean years.

If You Can't Grow It

It didn't take long before I began building my clientele. It was no longer clients just wanting to increase length and density; however, in addition, I began getting new clients who were starting to experience moderate hair thinning and hair loss. Their hair loss issues were noticeable. They didn't just want my services; they needed my services.

At that time, my business motto was, "If you can't grow it, I'll sew it and noone will know it". It was a true statement and something that I worked hard to provide to my clients. However, as the new clients sought my services, they presented more than creative styling sessions, and I realized the challenge ahead of me.

God Has a Sense of Humor

My mentor Rodney Barnett, Trichologist, always says, "When all you have is a hammer, everything looks like a nail." It would be many years later that I would have the opportunity to meet him, but I can truly say how true that statement was to me during that time.

All I had was a hammer, I could weave the heck into some hair. If you know anything about a hair weave, it's only as good as the foundation. Most importantly, the foundation keeps it anchored on. During that time the foundation was either a braid, interlocking foundation of hair, or something that required hair for stability. For 98% of these new clients with minimal hair loss and thinning, I was able to still provide a beautiful service for them.

However, for two percent (2%) of those remaining, what I noticed is that those clients required maintenance or "tightening" services more frequently than those clients without hair loss or thinning. Due to their thinning hair, I didn't realize what I know to be true now. Any type of extensions or hair weave services may cause traction and stress to the cuticle and scalp. Thus, clients with extremely fine, thinning hair may not be a good candidate for extensions and/or weave services. The last thing the stylist or client should want to do is add more weight to their hair with extensions if it is already too thin, short, and/or damaged.

What they should have been offered was a wig. However, I personally abhorred wigs. During my cosmetology training, I loathed Chapter 15 of Milady's Standard Textbook of Cosmetology, "The Artistry of Artificial Hair". God has a sense of humor. Who but He knew I would many years later learn to love, serve others, and change lives with wigs? During those years, they looked so "wiggy", artificial, and fake. I wasn't opposed like some people are to artificial hair. I was a "weave-ologist", I just hated anything that looked fake. Wigs during that time looked nothing like the innovative hair options of today. What's ironic is, my feelings now are weaves are similar to sewn-on wigs. I guess it's all about perspective.

Hindsight is 20/20

I wish I knew then, what I know now. As licensed professionals, our clients look to us to identify and provide the correct service, advice, and care to them. Even if that means referring them to a specialist. Just as in the medical profession, there are physicians who practice general medicine and there are those doctors who have spent additional time studying specialized medicine. It is the same in the beauty industry. There are licensed cosmetologists who are strictly general practitioners. Some are very adept at cutting and styling, others color, others provide perms, and others only braid hair. There are those who have chosen to study Trichology and hair loss. Ironically, there are those professionals that have not identified their limitations in certain areas, this may prove problematic for clients.

My rule of thumb, now as a seasoned professional is if I haven't been trained or certified in a specific discipline, I don't trust myself to offer it. There are services that I have trained and been certified to provide; however, they don't speak to me like offering specialized services for those clients living with hair loss.

We all have talents in some areas and limitations in others, that's nothing to be ashamed of. If you are a licensed stylist limited in an area of service, make sure you have resources of other professionals that can fill in those spaces. Network and align yourself with win-win opportunities. If you specialize in an area, offer incentives for referrals to stylists who do not offer those services.

Again, we're talking about many years ago, when I was still wet behind the ears when it came to my services. I just didn't want to turn away anyone needing my help. However, I have learned over time, there are some very legitimate occasions when a professional "No" is indeed warranted. Your client will inevitably appreciate it. In addition, have resources that you can refer them to. Now I have a network of other Trichologists, Hair Loss Practitioners, Hair Replacement Specialists, Dermatologists, Counseling Services, etc. to choose from. At that time, however, there were only a few reputable wig stores available and there were no hair loss professionals or Trichologists that I knew of in the area.

That Was Then This is Now

Now with everything easily accessible via the internet, mostly everything is virtually a Google Search away. If you are needing a specialist knowledgeable in hair and scalp maladies, consider seeking assistance from a certified Trichologist. Dermatologists can be very helpful when it comes to helping with hair loss and thinning as well; however, there are distinctive differences when it comes to both professions, discussed in a later chapter.

Whether you are seeking assistance as someone with hair loss or a licensed professional needing assistance for a client, there are legitimate help and resources out there. One specifically is a directory of Hair Loss Professionals, the "Hair Loss Pros Direct" App where you can find a hair loss professional in your area. For now, know there is help available.

As much as I am an advocate now for understanding hair loss and those affected by it, I thought it was important for you to understand a little about me; not the now me, but the me before today. My earliest and fondest memories revolve around hair and led me to a career that I love. My specialty, as it relates to helping clients with alopecia, was a work in progress. Like most things, it did not happen overnight. However, every client and every minute I have spent behind the chair prepared me for the writing of this book. My clients have shared some raw and emotional experiences, in distinct detail, that could not be healed without going through a process. Life is about processes. Especially with losing your hair.

* * *

For the Spirit God gave us does not make us timid, but gives us power, love and self-discipline. *2 Timothy 1:7 (NIV)*

CHAPTER 3

HAIR CYCLE AND HAIR LOSS

How It Develops

A lthough the process of hair development and loss may appear to be simplistic, it actually consists of three separate phases. These hair development stages have been examined in great detail. Age, nutrition, and general health can all have an impact on how quickly each phase progresses.

Anagen Phase

The anagen phase is the first stage of hair development. The hair on your head undergoes this phase for three (3) to five (5) years, yet for some people, a single hair may continue to grow for seven (7) or more years.

Fortunately, different hair types have different anagen phases. For instance, the anagen phase of pubic and brow hairs is significantly shorter than that of scalp hairs. Your hair follicles are releasing hairs during the anagen phase that will keep growing until they are trimmed or until they reach the end of their life cycle and fall out. Approximately 90% of the hairs on your head are in the anagen phase at any given time.

Catagen Phase

When the anagen phase concludes, the catagen phase begins and typically lasts 10 days or so. Hair follicles shrink and hair development slows down during this phase. The hair also breaks off from the base of the hair follicle, but it hangs on for a few more days as it grows. On average, just five percent (5%) of the hairs on your head are ever in the catagen phase.

Telogen Phase

Normally, the telogen period lasts three months. Approximately 10 to 15 percent of the hairs on your scalp are in this phase. During the telogen phase, hairs do not often develop or fall out. In follicles that have recently released hairs during the catagen phase, new hairs begin to form during the telogen phase.

Hair Loss

Simply put, alopecia means abnormal hair loss. Numerous situations, from those that compel people to pull their hair out, to the toxicity of chemotherapy for treating cancer, can all result in hair loss. While some causes are thought to be benign, others are warning signs of serious health issues. Some conditions are limited to the scalp, while others show the body's overall illness. The skin and its components can reveal early indicators of illness elsewhere in the body since they are so immediately apparent. Frequently, illnesses that affect the scalp's skin can cause hair loss.

Alopecia Types

Androgenic Alopecia, a genetic condition caused by the male hormone Dihydrotestosterone (DHT). DHT causes Male Pattern

Baldness in men and Female Pattern Baldness in women. This is the most common form of alopecia.

Alopecia Areata is an autoimmune disease in which the immune system attacks hair follicles at the root and causes hair to fall out. If not treated, it can advance to Alopecia Totalis or Alopecia Universalis.

Alopecia Totalis, a complete loss of hair on the scalp, is an inflammatory disease of the hair follicle. It is an advanced form of alopecia areata.

Alopecia Universalis is a complete loss of total body hair; including eyelashes, eyebrows, chest hair, leg hair, arm hair, armpit hair, and pubic hair. This is considered the most severe form of alopecia areata.

Telogen Effluvium, is a diffuse type of hair thinning that affects people after they experience severe stress or a change to their body. This is currently being seen in many people recovering from the coronavirus.

Central Centrifugal Cicatricial Alopecia, an unique form of scarring alopecia, usually causes permanent hair loss on the crown of the scalp, presented by inflammation. Inflammation causes Central Centrifugal Cicatricial Alopecia, but not Alopecia Totalis or Alopecia Universalis. Neither presents with scarring or redness, as the scalp is smooth and colorless.

Trichotillomania is a compulsive disorder, also known as a hair-pulling disorder. Hair can be pulled from anywhere on the body. See Trichotillomania (TTM Perspective).

Traction Alopecia, hair loss resulting from the continuous pulling force on the hair roots. Usually generated from tight styling methods like ponytails, braiding, etc., and can be prevented.

* * *

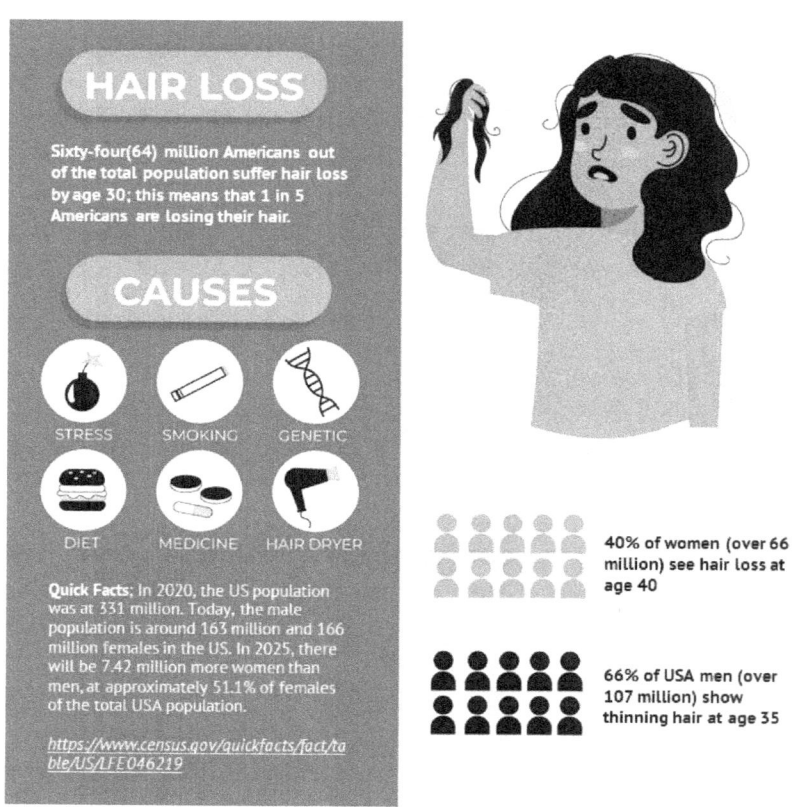

"Designed by Freepik"

Primary Causes of Hair Loss

Genetic Factors – Inherited Traits, Inflammation, Cystic Acne

Stress Inducing – Chronic, Traction, and Traumatic

Health Related – Illness, Low Vitamin Absorption, Hormones (Pregnancy, Menopause), Immune Disorders, Scarring/Burns,

Slow Circulatory System

Diet Concerns – Crash Diets, Nutritional Deficiencies, Excessive Vitamin A

Medical Issues – Birth Control Pills, Chemotherapy/Radiation Treatments, Hormonal Imbalance, Medications (Prescriptions)

Environmental Exposure – Photo Toxic Effect of the Sun, Air Pollutants, Employment Hazards, Water Chemical Levels

Hair Loss Stages

Hair Loss stages can be classified as a type of inherited hair loss called pattern baldness. It happens when the hair follicles have a genetic propensity to miniaturize or shrink, producing finer, weaker hair and eventually baldness. Both men and women can experience pattern hair loss, which is commonly referred to as male pattern hair loss and female pattern hair loss. However, certain types of pattern baldness may be more prevalent in one gender than the other.

* * *

Male Hair Loss Stages

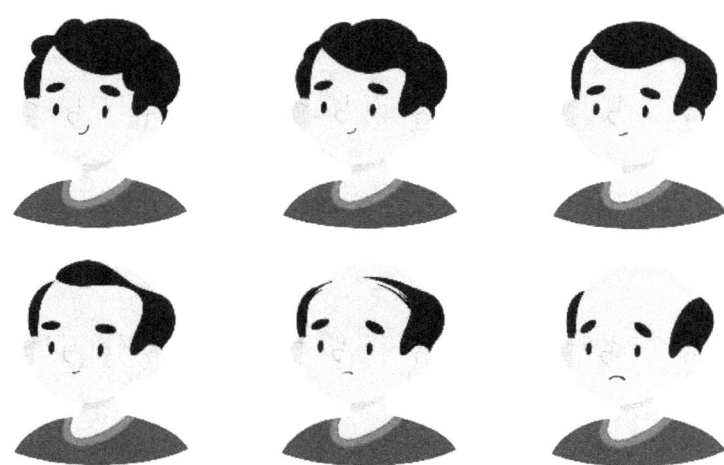

Female Hair Loss Stages

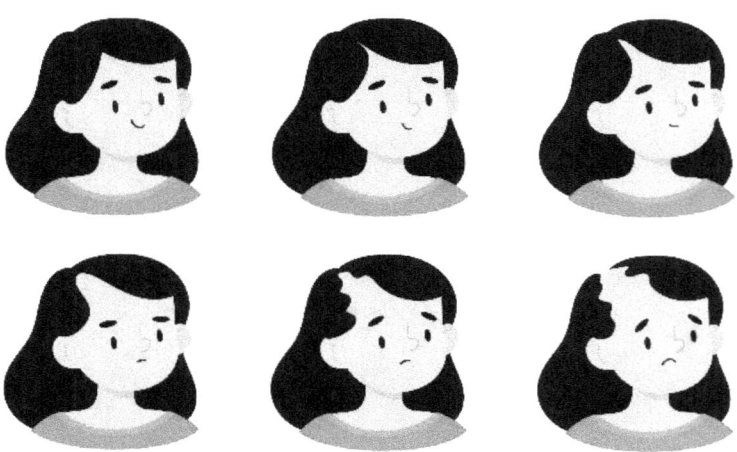

"Designed by pikisuperstar /Freepik"

Trichotillomania (TTM – Perspective)

For many people, hair is a statement piece; it is one of the most outwardly expressive projections of a person's identity. Whether the texture or style is straight, curly, coily, 3c, lower taper fade with designs, dreads, or even a beautiful bold bald scalp. What one does with their hair says something about who they are. Our hair is a part of our identity just as much as our name, smile, attire, personality, or sense of humor. Losing any part of our identity can be especially challenging, producing intrapersonal conflict.

So, what does happen when we lose a big part of our identity, like our hair, to a body-focused behavior like trichotillomania? "Trichotillomania (DSM-5-TR; American Psychiatric Association [APA], 2022) may be understood as a heroic unwillingness to completely submit to self-annihilating accommodation—a self-preserving compromise or defensive solution—requiring neither the relinquishment of self nor of attachment. It is the equivalent of using a code language to bypass the revelation of dangerous information" (Shumsky, 2013). Chronic hair-pulling (trichotillomania) is a nonfunctional habit (Snorrason et al., 2012) and can cause people to experience the following symptoms: symptoms parallel to the grief and loss journey, a decline in self-esteem, and essentially a loss of identity.

Denial, anger, bargaining, depression, and acceptance, are all stages of grief and are normal feelings associated with trichotillomania. When we consider grief and loss, typically thoughts of losing the physical being of a person comes to mind; or learning to live and adjust without a specific person. However, we can experience grief and loss, then continue physically carrying on. The death of any part of one's identity can be confusing, mentally exhaustive, and can produce negative self-talk triggering self-doubt and decreased compassion. Trichotillomania can be powered by internal intrusive thoughts, but the external implications are far more noticeable. Trichotillomania causes bald spots in places where hair was once abundant. During these anxiety-fueled and compulsive episodes (APA, 2022), an affected person does not consider the outcome of the episode; during this moment they feel more compelled to complete the compulsion despite any feelings warning them to stop.

During the hair-pulling episode, one may feel the release of tension, relaxation, or even happiness (Neal-Barnett & Stadulis, 2006). The affected person would experience a momentary positive outcome, but oftentimes the chain reaction of an episode would result in patches of bald spots. These spots are typically found in very noticeable areas visible to all; including on the head, eyebrows, arms, legs, and anywhere else hair can grow (APA, 2022). Since hair is often viewed as a statement piece, the residual effects of losing one's hair can be destructive to the self-image. Because of the visible reminders, people tend to experience complex feelings, going between self-blame, shame, fear, anger, and rejection. The trajectory of these feelings is comparable to the stages of grief and loss. Treatment for such disorders is best when tailored to the affected person, there is no "one-size fits all" approach. Everyone's journey and symptoms are unique, and their treatments should be also.

Individuals who are presented with trichotillomania tend to turn inward and place blame on themselves for their appearance. Once one can identify and work on triggers to hair-pulling, one can begin to decrease compulsive behaviors and the anxieties that drive the behavior (Snorrason et al., 2012). This process can be a tedious journey and the affected person should spend a fair amount of time finding the right person to help assist them in their therapeutic voyage. Find someone who will mindfully walk beside you, at your pace, and is willing to nurture all your feelings and emotions; while helping you improve on the new relationship you are developing with yourself (Homan & Hosack, 2019). If I have learned anything from my professional and personal experience with losing a part of my own identity, it is that showing yourself grace and self-compassion goes a long way.

Sasha Pinson, MS, LPC, NCC, Licensed Professional Counselor in San Antonio, Tx. Bachelor of Science in Psychology and Master's in Clinical Mental Health Counseling from the University of Texas in San Antonio

* * *

Male Pattern Baldness (MPB)

Moreover, hair recedes from the scalp in men with male pattern baldness (MPB), leaving a bald spot at the front of the head that resembles a horseshoe. Dihydrotestosterone (DHT), a male hormone, and genetics cause it to typically begin in early adulthood.

The most noticeable sign of male pattern hair loss is evident. Hair loss is the sign. Male pattern baldness can affect the top of their heads as well as their temples, where it may subtly spread to their eyebrows over time.

Each MPB patient will experience different symptoms. While some people's hair will thin out gradually until they are entirely bald on top, others will lose their hair quickly. The Hamilton-Norwood Scale is used to classify the stages of hair loss in men. The stages are described with a number from 1 to 7.

Female Pattern Baldness (FPB)

Female pattern baldness is the most typical kind of hair loss in women, as opposed to male pattern hair loss. Thinning hair, wider parts, and visible scalp result from hair loss, which happens while hair follicles are in their resting phase.

Also, it is hormonal resulting from the androgen Dihydrotestosterone (DHT) and genetics, female pattern baldness (FPB) in women is seen most often in hair loss clinics. Genetics, stress, and other medical issues are only a few of the potential causes.

About one-third of women suffer from female pattern baldness. Hair loss on the top or front of the scalp and a general decrease in hair density are two of the most typical signs. The Ludwig Scale is used to classify the stages of hair loss in women. The stages are described with a number from 1 to 3.

MPB attacks the hairline and can create a circular pattern in the vertex (crown). FPB generally doesn't attack the hairline, leaving it intact and creating an oval-type pattern directly behind the hairline.

Getting to the root of the "why" of losing hair helps one to understand causation. However, understanding the emotional impact of losing hair may or may not be fully understood. We do know, moreover, there are those who are starting to feel anxious as the issue slowly becomes worse. Finally, your hair stylist acknowledges that your hair is getting thinner. She suggests supplementing with vitamins, massaging your scalp, and destressing your life. Honestly, your life will not become any easier any time soon, despite the fact that you believe stress to be the likely culprit. Now when you are starting to get bald, you're scared. You identify with your hair; if you lose it, who are you?

Cancer and Losses

As the human body endures the rigors of chemotherapy and cancer treatment, numerous changes do take place. There are external changes as well as internal changes. The lady you see in the mirror will not be the "you" that you are familiar with or love. She has a different appearance, and her entire physique is changed. There is a good chance that you have put on or lost weight, forfeited some strength and stamina, and have a lot less energy than usual. These adjustments brought on by the chemotherapy typically seem insignificant in comparison to the baldness and loss of other body hairs. The most noticeable hair loss is on the head; but many women feel much worse about the lack of pubic hair, eyebrows, and eyelashes.

Although your oncologist may have forewarned you about hair loss, were you also ready for the emotional toll it would take? Why do I ask? Patients require emotional assistance as well. Being bald during chemotherapy is challenging, but being bald after chemotherapy is burdensome as well. Since losing hair is so widely connected with having cancer, everyone who has it is desperate to grow their hair back as soon as the treatment is through. Unfortunately, hair will grow on average half an inch per month.

Keep in mind that your body will not even be aware that your therapy is over for a while. No hair will regrow until your body has finished eliminating all of the chemotherapy cocktail's active chemical ingredients. Also, keep in mind that your hair grows from the inside of your scalp and takes time to appear as stubble. Six (6) to eight (8) weeks following the last session of chemotherapy, the majority of women see fuzz on their heads, this is frequently snow-white. Through 12 to 16 weeks after their final chemotherapy treatment, the majority of women do not feel confident removing their wigs, hats, or scarves.

It will probably take an extra four months or more, unless you kept your hair really short, to grow out enough hair to have the same or a comparable style before experiencing cancer.

Words I Had Never Heard Before

Celeste was early to her appointment with me that day. She is one of those "Early is on time, on time is late, and late is unacceptable!" type of clients. She was losing her hair; however, unlike most people, she knew why. It was only two weeks earlier that Celeste called to schedule her consultation. The phone call to make the consultation was unremarkable, general information was taken and contact information was asked of her to secure the appointed date and time. My front desk staff was instructed to be courteous, kind, and a listening ear but to not answer any questions regarding the diagnoses or specifics. More in-depth questions are asked during the actual consultation itself.

I had concluded my previous appointment 15 minutes prior and was preparing my office for my next client, Celeste. Intentionally allowing a few moments to not only "straighten up" physically, but spiritually and mentally as well. I always take a moment in between clients to gain perspective and clarity, seeking guidance to be able to assist each client that walks through my door. This client was no different.

At 2:00 PM precisely, Ms. Crawford, my front desk staff escorted Celeste into my office. Greeting her, I welcomed Celeste to take a seat. Once I sat behind my desk, I was able to review the notes from the Client Profile she filled out. At first glance, Celeste was an attractive woman in her mid-30s. Her occupation was in computer technology, she enjoyed reading and gardening in her spare time. It was easy to tell that she was nervous. My job was to make her feel comfortable and at ease. At this juncture in my career, if a client is coming to me, it has something to do with them losing their hair. This understandably would make anyone uncomfortable.

Breaking the ice, Celeste stated that she was recently married, had no children, and recently moved to San Antonio, TX, with her husband. San Antonio, TX, is known as "Military City USA" due to several military installations located within the city; a great percentage of my clients are military-connected. It was during a recent Well Woman exam at Wilford Hall Medical Center at Lackland A.F.B. that she was given her diagnosis, it was breast cancer. She mentioned that she routinely conducted monthly breast examinations. It was because of this routine during one month, she felt a small lump. She was not alarmed but decided to get it checked out. When the doctor told her she had breast cancer, they were proactive. Surgery was scheduled and subsequent chemotherapy. She was counseled on the high probability of losing her hair a couple of weeks after receiving treatment. That's why she called me, in anticipation of losing her hair.

There, I could feel it…her nervousness had gone. She was open and talking, sharing, and being encouraged. I began to learn more about her, then we decided on the best type of cranial prosthetic for her. She wanted a natural look. A wig that looked as close as possible to her "BEFORE" losing her hair look. I made measurements of her head, then we chose her hair color, texture, length, density, etc. I requested that she email me an inspiration photo for the type of look she wanted.

As I began to complete the notes of the consultation from the information gathered, it was then that she said it. Words I had never heard before during a consultation. Although it was the first time, it wasn't the last.

Celeste said, "Ms. Anderson, I have come to peace with having breast cancer. I am hopeful with the course of treatment I will be undergoing." I nodded as a sign of support. She then asked, "Do you know what the hardest part of it is?" Before I could answer, and I am glad I didn't; because I could never have guessed what she was about to say. She continued, "The hardest part is not having my breast removed. The hardest part is losing my hair." And a tear fell. As I handed her a tissue, I pondered my next words. If you know me, rarely am I at a loss for words. However,…this was a profound statement and sentiment that I had not heard before. Although I must admit at the time, I was somewhat dumbfounded by them. I respected Celeste's feelings.

As I opened my mouth to speak, (and at this moment of writing, I can't remember what responsible reply I had prepared) she spoke as she wiped away a tear, "I can't wait to see my new hair that you're getting for me."

"Of course, you can't, I promise not to make you wait any longer than necessary!" I exclaimed. I understood the assignment and I was confident that I could get her just what she asked for. Subsequently, the consultation was concluded.

It was three weeks afterwards that Ms. Celeste came in for her wig fitting. Her order was complete and ready. Her initial appointment had to be canceled and rescheduled. She wasn't feeling up to the visit following a recent chemotherapy session. However, this day, she was ready and so was her new hair. When she sat down, she removed her cap. It had started, her hair falling out from the chemotherapy. She asked if I would shave off her remaining hair. "I have cancer, it doesn't have me!" She confidently stated, "I am in control!" After finishing her shave-down, I fit the wig on her head, styled it, and showed her how to maintain it. She was excited when I handed her the mirror, and a small tear fell from her eye. It was when she looked at her reflection, she said, "I remember her". "Thank you, Jesus!" I thought to myself. I smiled.

Moments like that are priceless. It confirms to me the ministry I have chosen. It is more than a job. Celeste, however, wasn't the last client that said losing a breast was easier than losing their hair. It is another accounting that hair is a key part of our self-image and how important having it is.

Alopecia – Identifying

In my facility, clients come to me as I practice Trichology, seeking assistance with hair restoration and/or hair replacement. The latter, I specialize as a Non-Surgical Hair Replacement Specialist certified with a specialty in Medical Hair Loss.

Most times, these potential clients are seeking help after

consulting with, or prior treatment, from their Primary Care Physician or Dermatologist. My consultation is a very thorough process. It consists of the various methods listed above to determine the best option available to help the client. Treatment is as individual as the client, it is not "cookie-cutter"; however, as individual to the client the treatment plan may be, the consultation questions are the same. One of the most important questions I ask is: "Have you been diagnosed with Alopecia (hair loss)? If so, which type?" Many of those clients who answered "yes" could not identify the specific type(s) of Alopecia they were diagnosed with. That is where my expertise in Trichology comes in.

Abnormal Hair Loss

It is true, one client can have more than one type of Alopecia at one time. However, the term Alopecia means abnormal hair loss. There are different types of Alopecia, the main types include Alopecia Areata (AA), Alopecia Totalis (AT), Alopecia Universalis (AU), Androgenic Alopecia (AGA), Telogen Effluvium (TE), Anagen Effluvium (AE), Postpartum Alopecia, Central Centrifugal Cicatricial Alopecia (CCCA), Traction Alopecia (TA) and Trichotillomania (TTM).

Trichologists are paramedical professionals and do not diagnose medical conditions. However, we specialize in hair and scalp maladies and can identify varying types of Alopecia. Each form of Alopecia has specific traits and characteristics that make them easier to classify. Alopecia Areata (patchy) exhibits as one, multiple, separate, or conjoined smooth patches on the scalp. Alopecia Totalis is total hair loss on the scalp. Alopecia Universalis by definition is total hair loss on all areas of the body. Those are just a few examples of the visible and identifying differences of Alopecia.

Treating Hair Loss

The majority of hair loss cases have multiple underlying reasons, so a multi-therapeutic strategy is needed to effectively treat the issue. Therefore, in order to best treat your hair loss, the Trichologist will recommend the most advanced treatment approaches. The most asked question is, "Will it grow back?" There are so many factors that determine the hair's ability to grow. Depending on why you lost your hair, how long you have been losing it, age, hormones, heredity, etc., the list goes on, these will determine your chances of re-growth.

As a Trichologist, I would love to be able to grow back everyone's hair that comes to my facility. However, that's not the reality of life. The truth is not everyone's hair comes back fully. There are those who have significant amounts of their hair restored, while others experience minimal growth. Those whose hair doesn't grow back in its entirety have other options available to them.

Non-surgical Hair Replacement (NSHR) allows me the ability to provide that look of hair that many of my clients are looking for. I can't promise everyone that their hair will grow back; however, the promise of a beautiful, natural-looking head of hair via a cranial prosthesis hasn't failed me yet (knock on wood). For those who envision themselves as having hair once again, it's my go-to method of practically "instantaneous" hair. However, even NSHR isn't for every client.

Trichology, What Is It?

The paramedical science and study of hair, hair loss, and related scalp issues are known as Trichology. It includes research on conditions affecting the human scalp and hair, as well as evaluations of their causes and remedies.

The term "trichology" was first developed as a specialized field of study in Britain in the late 19th century and is derived from the Greek word "Trikhos," which means "hair." Then in 1902, it was given its para-medical specialty. Trichology is viewed as the "link between cosmetology and dermatology" in modern society.

Trichologists, What Do They Do?

A Trichologist is a paramedical (not a medical doctor) practitioner who is an expert in identifying and treating hair and scalp maladies. Since they are formally trained in the life sciences, they approach hair loss and scalp issues holistically by assessing clients based on their personal histories, lifestyles, genetic makeup, and environmental variables. A Trichologist can propose personalized treatment plans, nutritional guidance, and lifestyle adjustments based on this data to enhance the health, look, and quality of the hair and scalp.

Qualified Trichologists, like other paramedical (not medical doctors) specialists like dietitians, ayurvedic practitioners, phlebotomy technicians, etc. should collaborate closely with your medical doctor to determine whether any medical issues are connected to your hair loss. Additionally, your doctor should be open to doing and interpreting any blood tests that your Trichologist recommends, in conjunction with working with your Trichologist.

A proficient Trichologist ought to be able to relate to you on an empathic level. As part of your treatment plan, he or she should spend time giving you tips on how to manage your situation.

Difference Between Dermatologist and Trichologist

Have you thought about seeking professional advice about your scalp condition or hair loss? In that case, are you familiar with the distinctions between a Dermatologist and a Trichologist?

A Dermatologist specializes in skin conditions, whereas a Trichologist focuses on different types of Alopecia (hair loss), hair and scalp maladies. Additionally, a Trichologist collaborates with Medical Doctors, Internal Medicine Doctors, Endocrinologists, Neurologists, Psychologists, Nutritionists, Naturopathic Doctors, Dermatologists, Cosmetologists, and Barbers.

Alopecia treatments and therapies for scalp disorders should be combined with additional medical treatments and/or therapy for some systemic illnesses. There are a few significant comparisons noted below:

Dermatologist:

- Listens to the client for symptoms and indicators, but doesn't necessarily extensively inspect the scalp

- May administer scalp injections of steroids

- May recommend a biopsy

- May jot down a prescription

- Often advises the patient to halt all chemical reactions

Trichologist:

- Will discover the history of your alopecia and/or scalp issue

- Examines symptoms and signs

- Examines for pimples and lesions on the scalp

- Examines the skin for erythema and inflammation

- Examines for scaly scalp conditions

- Examines for damaged hair follicles and/or alopecia

- Will examine the health of the scalp and the hair bulb using microscopes

- Will assess any dietary inadequacies that may be related to the issue

Advantages of Trichology

People with problems with their hair or scalp commonly seek the assistance of Dermatologists and/or Trichologists. However, it's important to keep in mind the variations between the two disciplines when looking at these two specialists.

The distinction is that Trichology, by definition, is a discipline that only focuses on the hair and scalp. A Dermatologist is a physician who has had special training in diagnosing and treating patients with benign and malignant conditions affecting the skin, scalp, nails, and nearby mucous membranes.

This implies that while Trichologists only focus on the hair and scalp, Dermatologists primarily focus on the skin and all the serious disorders that come along with it.

Trichologists are professionals, specially trained usually with a history and knowledge of cosmetology. These professionals have studied and trained with specialized knowledge of hair and scalp maladies. Dermatologists are conventional medical doctors, and as such, they only use a small number of medicinal treatments, such as minoxidil, steroids, or antifungal creams. In an effort to determine the type of alopecia, a dermatologist may do a biopsy. Usually, this does not provide a solution for hair loss.

* * *

My flesh and my heart faileth; But God is the strength of my heart and my portion for ever. *Psalms 73:26 (ASV)*

CHAPTER 4

THE STIGMA OF HAIR LOSS

Alopecia in Women is Stigmatized

Alopecia is stigmatized in our society, particularly when it affects women, and this is shown in comparison to situations with men; however, the result is different based on gender. If you are a bald male, you can virtually go undetected, but if you are a woman, you become the center of attention. Children and adults alike frequently look surprised by seeing a woman with hair loss, despite it being "very common"; it is nonetheless challenging to comprehend and accept. People typically react with sympathy because they assume that a woman with alopecia could also be suffering from a more serious condition, like cancer.

In other instances, the stigma exists because the woman with alopecia does not adhere to the standards of beauty that have been created by society. Given that hair has long been connected with femininity and that losing it can cause anxiety and depression in women, it follows that hair loss has an emotional impact on women. Denial is frequently followed by bouts of anger and despair before acceptance sets in, allowing one to start living with alopecia and developing coping mechanisms.

Although hair loss may appear to be an innocuous condition with minimal to no physical side effects, its psychological effects can be very devastating. Hair loss can ruin your self-expression and self-confidence, both of which are crucial components of your self-image. This book is my attempt to bring attention to this dilemma by examining the illness, its causes, and any potential psychological effects in great detail. Hopefully, by doing so successfully, it will remove much of the stigma and shame surrounding those who are living with alopecia and open up a greater understanding to others that are unaffected by it. I aim to eradicate the negative B.S., Belief Systems of those who are very opinionated about the subject of hair loss in ways that are harmful and detrimental to themselves and others.

Men and women of all ages can have hair loss, which is a common dermatological problem. Several underlying diseases, which we mentioned briefly earlier, can lead to hair loss; but they rarely have any physically hazardous side effects. Less cranial cushioning and less protection from the sun's rays are the main functional issues associated with a reduced hair count. Itching and irritation of the scalp may also be linked to hair loss. Even if it has no effect on a person's physical health, hair loss can have serious psychological effects and a significantly lower quality of life.

The Impact of Hair Loss

A person's appearance might be impacted by hair loss. Losing eyebrows and eyelashes can have a significant impact because they are both defining characteristics of a person's look. Another disadvantage of hair loss is that society as a whole may occasionally perceive it as the victim's inability to meet the standards of physical beauty that we have come to expect in society.

The link between hair loss brought on by stressful events or experiences in life and the ensuing psychological effects might become more intricate. This difficulty may lead to more distress, worry, and despair. When compared to women who do not encounter as much stress, those who do have a hair loss problem are 10+ times more likely to do so.

People who have experienced the impacts of baldness are more prone to psychiatric illnesses than those who have not. Depression, anxiety, social phobias, and paranoid disorder are only a few examples of the psychological conditions that were mentioned above.

How Can Hair Loss Affect One's Mental Health?

There is little research on the psychological issues brought on by hair loss. While this is true, every day in my hair treatment facility I encounter many clients who openly share their feelings about losing their hair. The research demonstrates that experiencing hair loss is psychologically harmful, producing severe emotional pain and frequently resulting in issues with one's personal, social, and professional life. Psychological anguish is more likely to occur in those with severe hair loss than in those with modest hair loss. Hair loss might be interpreted as a failure to uphold social standards for physical beauty.

The Importance of Hair: Why?

Scalp hair contains a lot of symbolism; "healthy hair" is frequently linked to perceptions of attractiveness, charm, beauty, class, and power. Hair can also convey information about social standing and cultural origin. For instance, observant Jewish males wear the traditional sidelocks (Payot) to signal status among their peers, and monks often shave their heads. Rastafarians, also known as rastas, grow dreadlocks; nor do they cut their hair because it is where their strength lies.

Making sure your hair is styled for the day is a crucial step in getting ready to face the outside world. So, what happens if your hair starts thinning and you are no longer in control of the social cues it sends? The phrase "bad hair day" is a reminder of the psychological significance of hair; hair loss can make every day a bad hair day.

The Blessing and Curse

To keep up with current trends in our fashion-conscious society, it seems we are willing to do virtually anything to our hair. We submit our hair to a number of demanding routines every day; including thermal styling, flat irons, weaving, perming, coloring, and braiding.

However, taking care of hair needs close attention to detail. While "looking beautiful" is a valid concern, a greater one should be developing a true understanding of our hair and its requirements in order for it to stay strong and healthy.

God gave our hair texture as a gift, not a curse. The hair of Black women is among the most adaptable in the world. Its thick, coarse texture makes sure that we are well-protected from the elements; it has been placed on our heads to do so. We may style it in a variety of ways, including straight, wavy, curly, cornrowed, twisted, and loc'd. We are lovely and distinctive due to a variety of things, including our adaptability and creative range. Ironically though, this talent for adaptability has turned into the cause of many black women's hair issues. Black women frequently experiment more with hair products and styles since there are so many options available to us, occasionally not in our favor.

Over the years, I have provided my professional services to many clients who detailed the many different styles which eventually resulted in Traction Alopecia (TA). It has never been my intention to blame anyone for a self-inflicted illness or lifestyle-related disease.

The Blame Game

We must address the moral implications of taking personal responsibility for sustaining our health. The environment, economics, and genetics are all factors that affect health in addition to one's own actions, and it can be challenging to establish a link between the three.

Self-inflicted illnesses brought on by drunkenness, drug addiction, obesity, and even lung cancer (if not contracted by second-hand smoke) are sometimes stigmatized and blamed on the person. Many people think those who are afflicted deserve our wrath since they brought it on themselves. Or in the case of Traction Alopecia (TA), they should be made fun of.

Please, humor me, in this analogy. No, I haven't lost my mind. I realize that drunkenness may eventually lead to cirrhosis of the liver and subsequently death. Drug addiction could result in an overdose and loss of life. Obesity could lead to a myriad of health crises including hypertension, diabetes, stroke, etc., and possibly even death. Smoking can lead to cardiovascular and respiratory diseases, lung cancer, etc., and yes, loss of life. The common denominator in a worst-case scenario for each of these activities is an untimely death. It's true, no one has died from Alopecia even though many times it's a serious immunological disease. Some people continue to view it as a purely aesthetic issue.

Due to this stigma and the reality that alopecia doesn't truly affect a patient's life expectancy, alopecia has not been given high priority for research. This disregard for alopecia has been shown by the medical sector and has permeated into the general public. There's not a lot of understanding or compassion; that's why many people suffer from alopecia in secrecy.

Traction (or Traumatic) Alopecia (TA)

By overusing harsh chemicals like relaxers, permanent hair color, curly perms, and bleaches, this type of alopecia is self-inflicted. That's different from being intentional. Just meaning the causation being other than natural, hereditary, etc. The misuse of such harsh hair chemicals can also lead to hair breakage. But unlike breaking, which happens gradually and may eventually regrow, in traction alopecia, the hair breaks all at once and will not regrow.

Excessive tension along the hairline from tight braids, weaves or ponytails, is another factor in traction alopecia. The scalp becomes inflamed and eventually scarred because of continual pulling of the hair, eventually ripping it out of the follicle. Hair will not grow out of a scarred follicle on the scalp ever again. It's time to change your hairstyle if your scalp has any bumps or inflammation.

Traction alopecia is a condition that many people believe only black women are susceptible to. Traction alopecia can afflict women of all races and hair types; it is usually more frequently observed in those with afro-textured hair.

The prevalence of hair extensions has increased the number of Caucasian women who are affected, typically with patches of hair loss where the extensions have been placed in addition to the traction alopecia's trademark receding hairline. If tightly braided hairstyles become very popular, it's possible that more women will start to notice hair loss around their hairlines. This will happen if braids are worn too frequently.

Both sexes can be affected by traction alopecia; however, men tend to experience it less frequently because women prefer to experiment more with their hairstyles. Males can still lose their edges; however, it's more likely that this is because of a receding hairline brought on by male-pattern baldness.

It's No Laughing Matter

In order to understand this section of the book, I will have to take a little time to clarify a little terminology. An individual's hair in the forehead area naturally forms a border known as the hairline. The front hairline is another term for this area of the head. The word "edges" is widely used in the Black community to describe the front hairline. So, front "hairline" and "edges" may be used interchangeably.

Please don't hold me to the exact year, but I'm pretty sure I first watched this video back in 2015, though I could be wrong. The "Save My Edges" campaign was a parody "Public Service Announcement" video lineup which included a variety of celebrities.

In order to combat this "dreadful problem," they urged the audience to "take the pledge". We must do it for our "sisters, moms, daughters, aunties... the babies, baby hairs" and "to protect what is so very precious in our community...our edges." The "campaign" directs you to savemyedges.org, a CentricTV advertising website.

Well, I am not too proud to admit...after the 1st, 2nd, 3rd, viewing of the video, I was not at all amused. At first, I felt that it was irresponsible of the featured celebrities to utilize their notoriety and platform to make light of a delicate matter like hair loss. Particularly and especially Traction Alopecia (TA), which causes hair loss around the hairline, or "edges".

Traction alopecia is a condition that many people believe only black women are susceptible to. I concluded the phrase "protecting our community" was used in jest in the film, along with "saving our sisters, moms, daughters, aunts," and "save the babies" (pun intended) baby hairs.

Hair loss of any kind is NOT funny. Because I work with so many ladies living with hair loss, it is such a sensitive subject. Some of them may have even engaged in various forms of hair manipulation/styling; this eventually resulted in irreparable harm to their hair. More notably, their "edges" vanished before coming to me for assistance.

Many of these clients were paying braiders, who were braiding way too tightly. Women were sitting in other stylists' chairs for marathon weave sessions, where too much tension was being put on their tresses, eventually pulling them out. Attaching lace front wigs to their hairline with glues, adhesives, and/or tapes. Now, admittedly there were some clients who styled their own hair, never understanding that "catching up" the hairline and braiding it too tightly was the beginning of their own nightmare. They knew just enough, unfortunately, to be dangerous. Whether it was done by someone else or self-inflicted, the damage was done—it is unrecoverable and it is not laughable.

I was showing this video to a coworker, who likewise focuses on helping customers who are experiencing hair loss. She too was horrified. She inquired if I had heard the song about a girl without any edges—really? There is also a song. I'll never understand why we like making fun of other people's suffering. What I do know is that most people do not jest or laugh when they hear that someone has been diagnosed with cancer. Why? Because this person could succumb to the sickness based on a number of factors. Unlike cancer, as it turns out, people don't actually die from losing their hair. That fact does not make it less devastating. However, because alopecia removed the one thing they identified with, their hair, I have encountered numerous people who have quietly retreated emotionally within themselves; a form of "death". These people were never the same again. I digress...

Many of the comments on the video were full of mockery, making cruel jokes and poking fun at the video. There were pledges to commit to the PSA campaign. However, there were some that expressed their sadness; they like me, couldn't believe the PSA was real—which it was not. Others identified with the hair loss and wished they had help. Yes, it made me sad.

PSA – An Edge-ucational Effort

As I prepared for the writing of this book, I contemplated adding information about the tongue-in-cheek PSA from way back when. I decided to see if I could find it, I Googled it and went to the SaveYourEdges.org website (which is no longer up). I did some backward searches and finally decided to check out YouTube. It's true...EVERYTHING is on YouTube.

There it was, the video. Again, in all its transparency, it elicited the same emotion I felt when I saw it for the very first time. However, during my search, I found an article, a separate independent article. The article initially began to applaud the PSA and called it a funny spoof. However, as I began to read it, it began to paint a different picture of the intent of the video and the campaign #SaveMyEdges, as it was created back then.

In the PSA for the #SaveMyEdges campaign, ladies are urged to visit the website. The site detailed the various hairstyling methods that could result in hair loss and offered "edge-ucational" resources for preventing and treating Traction Alopecia.

The treatment for traction alopecia is not covered on this promotional site, despite the fact that it includes many helpful haircare tips for dealing with the condition of the hair on a cosmetic level. There were suggestions such as wearing the hair naturally, using castor oil to soften the hair, utilizing silk pillowcases or wearing silk headscarves to protect hair.

OK, why did I get so offended? It was a parody...am I too close to the situation to find humor in it? Why did they choose that medium to deliver their message? Well, maybe because they are in the entertainment industry. The "helpful" information on the website scratched the surface and was merely superficial on the "what to do"; but they are not in the profession that I am in. I see the pain in my client's faces, hear it in their voices, and feel it in the spirit of those clients who are living with hair loss. The entertainers do not, so it is to be expected that even though their intentions were to bring attention to a serious situation in a funny entertaining way, it still caused some people who left comments on the video to make inflammatory statements. Others felt the hurt as they too were living with hair loss. Why? Because it is emotional.

The Slap Heard Around the World

After the LIVE broadcast and for some time thereafter, all talk was about Jada Pinkett-Smith, whose alopecia was the punchline of a joke at the 2022 Oscars. Were you watching LIVE or did you hear about it later? If you're one of a few that hadn't heard about it, I want to know one thing...What?! Have you been hiding under a rock? How are you oblivious to the smack that was heard around the world?

So, this is what took place. Chris Rock, comedian, and presenter at the 94th Annual Academy Awards joked about Jada Pinkett Smith's hair loss by suggesting that she be chosen to play G.I. Jane in a film. Pinkett-Smith's husband, the actor Will Smith, stormed the stage in response and hit Rock in the face. Who, in your opinion, was more at fault?

Discussion of the event went on for days, weeks, and months. The event was polarizing. Practically everyone had an opinion.

Regardless of what side of the opinion you are on, I will share this. Although I do not condone violence and am unclear at what point teasing and making fun of those experiencing hair loss became socially acceptable—hair loss is no laughing matter.

From Smith's perspective, I would imagine watching someone you love begin to lose all of their hair and not being able to do anything about it is an agonizing process; and no one deserves to be made fun of for it. It is just as bad as any other form of body shaming, people who do it should be called out on it. If you think making fun of people who are fat, skinny, small, big, etc. is bad, but making fun of bald people is okay, then you are a hypocrite. Things could and should have been handled differently that evening. I have personal, real-time experiences of supporting clients as they work through the pain of living with hair loss.

The next day, Smith apologized directly to Rock in a public statement issued by his publicist and posted to Instagram.

"Violence in all of its forms is poisonous and destructive. My behavior at last night's Academy Awards was unacceptable and inexcusable. Jokes at my expense are a part of the job, but a joke about Jada's medical condition was too much for me to bear and I reacted emotionally.

I would like to publicly apologize to you, Chris. I was out of line and I was wrong. I am embarrassed and my actions were not indicative of the man I want to be. There is no place for violence in a world of love and kindness.

I would also like to apologize to the Academy, the producers of the show, all the attendees, and everyone watching around the world. I would like to apologize to the Williams Family and my King Richard Family. I deeply regret that my behavior has stained what has been an otherwise gorgeous journey for all of us."

Regardless of whether or not you have an opinion about this incident or not, that's okay. I would ask that you insert yourself into the shoes of any one of these people. Dismiss the fact they're celebrities, although celebrities are people too. What if it were the subject of anyone (Chris Rock) making the joke, at the expense of the subject (Jada Pinkett-Smith) of the joke, or the person (Will Smith) that escalated the joke? Ask yourself, what would you do and why? If you had an opinion before reading this book, has it changed, and if so, why? If not, why? Regardless of how you feel about it, it's always good to consider all perspectives of a situation.

Don't Make Fun of Bald People

The fact that losing your hair is not funny cannot be emphasized enough, in my opinion. Never mock bald folks; it's not cool. It might have disastrous effects to make fun of others. This Bible story truly epitomizes why it's not a good thing to ever belittle or bully anyone. Before I ever imagined this stage of my profession where I focus on offering services to clients who have hair loss, I had a childhood recollection. My parents trained my siblings and me to be considerate and courteous of everyone, regardless of who they are, what they have, or what they looked like.

I have read various Bible scholars' accounts of the true interpretation of the scriptures I am about to share. Meaning, there were additional reasonings on the what, when, and how. Those of us that read and study The Bible do understand this. However, I am going to just invite you to consider the following at face value. Just as the scripture reads, just like I did those many years ago as a child; At face value, the story is simple.

We studied about the prophet Elisha as young children in Sunday School (2 Kings 2:23-24). They laughed at Elisha. Young men from the town came out and made fun of the prophet as he traveled up to Bethel, shouting, "Get out of here, baldy!" Elisha turned around and looked at them, cursing them in the name of the Lord. Two female bears came out of the woods and mauled forty-two of the boys. End of story.

If that's not a viable case for practicing kindness, I don't know what is. Regardless of being slapped LIVE on stage in front of millions of people during prime time, being mauled by bears, or the many things that can happen in between... just remember, don't make fun of bald people.

In today's time, it is highly doubtful that you will meet the fate of those young boys who mocked the prophet, Elisha. However, I do believe that we reap what we sow. I simply believe that we all have to eventually face up to the consequences of our actions. It is much easier to live a nice peaceful life by being polite rather than by being rude and insolent.

Crude Words

Recently, I visited a forum on hair loss. The discussion topic was concerning crude and annoying things people say to others losing their hair. As we know, "words have power". Proverbs 18:21 (NIV) "The tongue has the power of life and death..." Many of the things shared by the members of the forum were hurtful and inconsiderate.

Here are a few of the comments shared: (HairLossTalk.com/ interact annoying-things-people-say-about-hair-loss)

- "It's only hair, get over it."

- "Hair loss is worse for someone who is 18 than someone in their 30s or 40s."

- "Worrying about hair loss is pure vanity."

- "There are people with things a lot worse than hair loss, stop being a baby!"

- "Losing your hair? That's because you need to take better care of your hair; stop being so lazy about it!"

- "You're losing your hair because you have a poor diet. Eat better, eat healthier!"

- "You don't take good enough care of yourself; that's why you're losing your hair!"

Many people feel driven to express any fleeting emotion, idea, or thought. Without considering the impact of what they are saying, they ramble off whatever is on their minds. Our focus is lost when we chat about unimportant things, such as other people.

Other people's words have meaning. Both the opinions of those closest to us and total strangers are important to us. And if we allow it, the things others say to us and about us can hurt. However, you have the choice not to let such statements have an impact on you. This is what I meant by other esteeming. When we value ourselves based on the opinions of others or anything else outside of ourselves, we are engaging in "other esteeming." Those who value themselves based on the approval of others are more vulnerable to experiencing low self-esteem in the face of rejection or failure.

Sticks and Stones

Words hurt, despite what the classic "sticks and stones" adage may have taught you. We are impacted by what other people say because we dislike being judged; as a result, we continuously worry about what others may think and say about us. We take great care to meticulously craft the image we want to present to the world. We all have various ideas, views, and values as humans; we invariably come into contact with people who have different viewpoints throughout our lifetimes. You must not worry about what other people think of you, especially in regard to you losing your hair. Too much concern for what other people think can make you feel powerless, ruin your day, or prevent you from being the best version of yourself.

* * *

I can do all things through Christ which strengtheneth me. *Phillipians 4:13 (KJV)*

CHAPTER 5

HOW HAIR LOSS IS FELT

Self-Image and Hair Loss

T he foundation of human personality and conduct is the "self-image." If you alter your self-perception, you will also alter your personality and behavior. What is self-esteem? It plays a crucial role in how we regard ourselves and determine our own value. It also directs how we connect with others and the world around us on a daily basis.

Numerous variables define self-esteem, including:

- Self-confidence

- Identity perception

- A sense of safety

- Feelings of confidence

- A sense of community

In general, childhood is when we have the lowest levels of self-esteem. As we become older, learn more about ourselves, and gain greater assurance in our ability to navigate the world, it gradually rises. However, in response to life events, self-esteem can go through sharp drops as well as sharp boosts.

Hair loss is a typical life experience that lowers self-esteem. Although hair loss is quite frequent and natural (50% of men experience hair loss by the age of 50), the experience can have a detrimental effect on self-esteem, which can impair behavior and confidence in social circumstances. In this book, we'll look at the connection between hair loss and self-esteem.

For centuries, and possibly even longer, hair loss has been associated with low self-esteem. Long, thick hair was once a representation of vigor, youth, health, and femininity. The contrary was also true; thinning hair hinted at the aging process. It is not surprising that, whether consciously or unconsciously, individuals continue to equate hair quality, thickness, and length with these aspects in today's image-focused world.

While I cannot speak for the people of ancient times, hair loss, balding, or thinning hair frequently causes emotions of anxiety, low self-esteem, and stress in modern men and women. In fact, a number of studies have established a link between male pattern hair loss (Androgenic Alopecia) and diminished confidence and self-esteem. In a *2005 study, researchers called a sample of men (*most studies are conducted on men rather than women) and inquired about their hair loss. Sixty-two percent (62%) of the men who had baldness agreed that it had a negative impact on their self-esteem. Of those surveyed, forty-three percent (43%) mentioned worries about how losing their hair would influence their appearance, forty-two percent (42%) possessed dread of being completely bald, thirty-seven percent (37%) worried about getting older, twenty-two percent (22%) experienced a decline in social life, and twenty-one percent (21%) had feelings of despair.

According to a 2019 study published in the International Journal of Trichology, androgenic alopecia, often referred to as male-pattern baldness or female-pattern baldness, has also been linked to a lower quality of life because of how people perceived themselves and conduct their interpersonal relationships. Even though these research findings highlight the difficulties experienced by those who have hair loss, that does not mean there are not any potential treatments.

How Low Self-Esteem Affects You

We now understand that losing one's hair might result in low self-esteem. But for those who live with it, what does that actually entail on a daily basis? There are several ways that low self-esteem can appear. Those who have poor self-esteem as a result of hair loss may:

- Refuse to go out with friends out of concern for how their hair will be perceived

- Possess negative and irrational thoughts, such as the notion that others are superior to them or that they are more attractive

- Feel ashamed discussing their hair and their feelings about it

- Concentrate too much on how their hair looks, which can be distracting from daily life

- Feelings of helplessness and lack of control over the future and their looks, as well as anxiety, self-doubt, and worry

- Having trouble with confidence in general

A range of mental health conditions, such as anxiety or depressive disorders, could potentially be brought on by low self-esteem. The effects of poor self-esteem are never pleasant, whether it is declining a fun dinner date, taking an eternity to find the ideal hat, or wasting money on pricey styling products. I will share strategies to boost low self-esteem caused by hair loss in the following paragraphs.

Increasing Self-Esteem

The good news is that hair loss is most definitely not fatal. There are several options available to those going through this, ranging from surgical procedures to non-surgical solutions. What are the major actions you can take to increase your self-esteem, then?

Yes, losing your hair may feel awful. Most of the time, it's not harmful. It can be easier for you to view hair loss as a psychological obstacle to conquer if you are aware that the physical changes to your body are not in any way life-threatening. This psychological difficulty can be overcome by discussing it with friends and family.

You may wish to modify your hairdo if your hair loss is apparent with shorter haircuts that can readily conceal thinning hair, hair loss is generally less obvious. Or you could consider wig options.

There are several reliable solutions at your disposal. Finding the best solution for you is all it takes to take charge of your hair, or lack thereof. I recommend contacting a Trichologist or Hair Replacement Specialist if you are suffering from both hair loss and low self-esteem. They will provide you with a consultation during which they will go through your options and recommend the best course of action.

Nowhere to Hide (Celebrity)

There is a natural curiosity for many when it comes to celebrities or famous people. Celebrity watching can be found everywhere, from Hollywood red-carpet events to the tabloids crowding the grocery checkout lines. Even the most laid-back person could find themselves browsing through a slideshow of "Red Carpet" attire following any major celebrity event. So why are celebrities so appealing to us?

It's absolutely normal most of the time. According to psychologists, humans are social animals that evolved in societies where it was advantageous to pay attention to those in positions of high standing. This inclination may have grown into celebrity attraction, which has been fostered by the media and technology.

Celebrity curiosity is so common in our society that there is a means to gauge how deep it goes. For some people, superstars have a drug-like effect. They surround us everywhere and because of that, for some, they are an easy "fix". This inclination is used by celebrities and the media. On websites like Twitter, celebrities interact directly with fans, offer interviews, and divulge juicy details about their personal lives. As a result, it's simpler than ever to engage in "parasocial" connections, the psychological term for the type of one-sided relationships people have with celebrities.

Sense of Style and Glitz

The personalities of celebrities are endearing. Their dazzling fashions have a profound impact on individuals. The law of nature dictates that well-known people or celebrities become brands and signatures in a certain community or throughout the entire globe.

As a result of their fame, people mimic their fashion choices. We've all seen renowned people, social icons, and influencers whose distinctive fashions others like copying for various occasions throughout their lives. Celebrities thrill people, and they enjoy emulating their fashion choices. Hollywood actors and actresses are well-known throughout the world, not just in the United States, and are frequently cited as the source of hair, makeup, fashion, beauty, and clothing trends. Fans love their favorite celebrities without condition. Or is that truly the case?

More Common Than You Think!

Everyone wants to appear their best, especially prominent people and celebrities. So, what happens when those full, gorgeous heads of hair begin to thin out and lose hair due to androgenic alopecia (male or female patterned baldness)? Some people elect to use shaving razors, while others decide to use wigs, toupees, and hair transplant surgery. Some people choose to accept the hair they have, or don't have.

It is fact, celebrities are real people too. It can be challenging to consider the famous as actual people at times. Their lives are so lavish, whereas ours are just routine. We must keep in mind that they are also human beings. Like us, they experience real emotions and deal with real issues. Including hair loss and seemingly how they react and deal with it depending on the individual. Just like it does with those of us who are not famous. In this section, we are looking at a few celebrities who have publicly discussed their hair loss. Other bald celebrities, without respect to their reasons, are rocking the look, and others don't have hair loss but have been "Balderized" (computerized editing) to give the appearance of hair loss.

Ask yourself, if seeing your favorite celebrity with hair loss changes your perception of them. Do you see them as anything less than before: less attractive, less smart, less professional, less gifted, less influential, less _____ (you fill in the blank), etc?

Picture of Perfection

I will try to prove the misconception and how it manifests, only because I believe society accepts baldness from men more readily than from women. Here is my disclaimer (because I just might be biased)...I love the look of a man with a bald head. Growing up, I remember more of my handsome father without hair than with it. My best friend, and eventual husband, confidently rocked a fully shaven head from the first night we met.

Over the years, however, many notable men have been quite reluctant to show their thinning hair and vanishing hairlines. Yet it seems that when they decided to go bald or to embrace it, people responded to them differently than they did to their female counterparts.

Boris Kodjoe, Bruce Willis, and Samuel L. Jackson all look good with bald heads. However, not every celebrity feels the same way about their thinning hair and receding hairlines. Sometimes it takes them a few or many years to accept their hair-free state. It is rumored that the signature high-top fade haircut of comedian/host Steve Harvey, that he was well known for, was actually a hairpiece. The actor Robert Pattinson revealed in an interview that he used a hairpiece in the final Twilight Movie. Tennis phenom, Andre Agassi can be added to the list. Impressively, his iconic '80s hair was a hairpiece. That makes his game performances even more outstanding.

The appearance of many other well-known figures, in my opinion, were improved by shaving. Notably, Damon Wayans, Jason Statham, Dwayne Johnson (better known as "The Rock"), and Vin Diesel, all look significantly better now that they embraced a clean-shaven appearance. Some of these actors have taken a trip on the Schick Razor Train, but others seem to be clinging to what's left of their once-flowing tresses.

When examining celebrity hair loss, it becomes clear that Michael Jordan has done more for bald guys than anybody else. The legendary international superstar is equally well-known for his bald head, as well as for his deity-like performances on the basketball court.

Who is Our Michael Jordan?

It's embarrassing to view my early videos, but this subject is of such importance that I don't mind digging into the vault of old videos. Because even before this book, this subject matter mattered to me.

Here's the excerpt from my original blog: trinitylacewigs. blogspot.com (TrinityLacewigs.Com (TLC) – Blogger)

Post – Dec 13, 2017 "Who is our Michael Jordan?"

"I know no one dies from hair loss, but it is life-changing; and the change most times than NOT isn't for the better. However, the appearance-related effects of hair loss can be devastating to anyone, ESPECIALLY women.

If offering Michael Jordan as a poster child for endorsing the acceptance of balding men...then who is the Michael Jordan for women?

(Video Transcript – Dec 2017)

0:09
Some time ago I ran across an archived article found in the November 2002

0:16
Journal of the Harvard Men's Health Watch. Now, in this article, a medical

0:22

doctor wrote about the different treatments that are available for hair

0:25

loss in men. And in this report, he mentioned the pros and the cons of the

0:31

treatments and concluded his opinions like this, and I quote, "From a medical

0:38

point of view, there is no need to treat normal hair loss. At best, the treatments

0:43

are only partially effective; and although they are generally safe, some

0:49

men may experience side effects. Take a look at the mirror and think it over and

0:55

before you decide to try, imagine how Michael Jordan would look with a bit of

1:01

hair." STOP THE PRESSES! Hi, my name is Stephanie Anderson from StephanieL

1:11

Anderson.com. Just please share, subscribe and like my channel. OK, so with

1:19

all that being said, this brings me to today's discussion. And if you've ever

1:25

heard me or seen me before, you really know that I am very quick to share,

1:30

because I believe that sharing is caring. I give statistical information and

1:36

really huge numbers; like many women in the United States are suffering from

1:42

hair loss. And the number is like 30 million. And yes, that's just the number of

1:49

cases reported on hair loss. Not just thinning, but discernible, visible hair

1:56

loss; which is roughly one out of every four women, everyday, are suffering

2:04

alone and in silence. Well, it's been my mission since 2009 to help bring a voice

2:11

to these women's hair loss that is considered a taboo.

2:15

It's shameful, it has a stigma associated with it, which only compounds the

2:22

helplessness and insecurity that many women are faced with. With so many

2:29

concerns in The World, someone may just ask, "What's the big deal? It's only hair!

2:35

Just put on a wig!" And you believe the cavalier, nonsensical (is that even a word?)

2:43

and insensitive comments, and retorts that I have heard over the years from

2:50

people and even professionals that I have tried to enlist in my quest to help

2:56

other women. Now, I don't believe that you personally have to experience hair

3:02

loss for yourself, to be able to feel for any woman who may be facing it. It just

3:10

happens to be that over the years, I have been fortunate enough and blessed to

3:16

train, to specialize in providing services to this special demographic of

3:22

clients. And not only provide services to them, but in ear and hopefully a voice

3:29

of support and to answer the asinine question as to, "It's only hair!" Well, let

3:38

me tell you this, it's only hair when you find yourself with not being faced

3:43

without it! Hair loss is not normal, and a lot of women have spent thousands of

3:49

dollars seeing doctor after doctor after doctor, many times receiving conflicting

3:57

diagnoses. Many spend more money on topical solutions and treatments and

4:03

shampoos, vitamins, herbal supplements, therapeutic devices, and so on, and so on.

4:10

They hold the implied promise of thicker, fuller, growing hair or enhancements. Now,

4:18

I know better than anyone that no one dies from hair loss, but it is life

4:23

changing. And the chance, most times

4:26

than not, for the better. My clients range from pubescent teens to seniors. And in

4:34

this stage of my professional career, I can honestly say that hair loss seems

4:39

relatively to not being a respecter of age, or race, or social economics, or

4:46

background. Now, I have counseled and serviced so many women, and it is

4:52

heart-wrenching the toll hair loss can take on a woman. It's very

4:57

devastating because many women feel ignored. They feel alone and helpless. It

5:03

can affect their self-esteem, which trickles down to how they respond at work

5:08

professionally with their bosses or co-workers or customers. It affects in their

5:13

personal lives with their spouses or significant others; and maybe with their

5:18

children, and even other family members. So with the article that I just read, if

5:24

you have a medical professional with the opinion that natural hair loss should

5:28

not be treated. Just imagine Michael Jordan with a bit of hair. Then riddle me

5:35

this…who is our Michael Jordan? Who will

5:40

represent the standard of balding women to the world? Just

5:45

take a look at these pictures and just imagine

5:56

all beautiful women. Yes, but it's not for everyone.

6:01

Listen, if you're a suffering with hair loss, feel free to contact me at info@

6:07

Stephanie L Anderson.com I am a certified holistic trichologist and I

6:14

utilize remedies and treatments that can help you; to restore your crown or

6:18

your hair. And if you're not in the San Antonio Texas area, no problem. Ask me how

6:25

we can schedule a no-obligation online consultation. That's info@

6:33

StephanieLAnderson.com. And come back here often for more information. What do

6:39

you have to lose, but more hair? Feel free to like, share, and subscribe to my

6:44

channel here on YouTube. Until next time, be blessed and goodbye!

It's 2022 – We Have a Dream Team

It shouldn't be considered taboo to talk about hair loss, especially in women. Over 21 million women in the United States alone are hair-loss sufferers. It's encouraging to see that some of our favorite celebrities are breaking conventions and starting the dialogue for us. Let's take a look at some of these courageous women:

Ricki Lake (an American television host and actress) – Ricki Lake is familiar with the psychological and emotional toll that hair loss can take. In 2020, Lake spoke candidly with Robin Roberts of "Good Morning America" about her ongoing battle with alopecia. Since then, Ricki has made her rounds on talk shows, podcasts, and other appearances, sharing her experiences. She also courageously made lengthy posts to social media, describing it as, "debilitating, embarrassing, painful, scary, depressing, lonely"—all these negative adjectives. Her hair loss journey began while playing the role of Tracy Turnblad in the 1998 movie, "Hairspray". Lake said that having her hair triple-processed and teased every day of filming meant her natural hair "was never the same". Since then, Lake said factors like, 'yo-yo dieting, hormonal birth control, radical weight fluctuations over the years, her pregnancies, genetics, stress, and hair dyes and extensions have caused significant hair loss.

Opening up about her struggles and posting pictures without a wig or extensions has a greater purpose. "I know that by sharing my truth, I will be striking a chord with so, so many women and men". She also confessed, "There have been a few times where I have even felt suicidal over it. Almost no one in my life knew the level of deep pain and trauma I was experiencing. Not even my therapists over the years knew my truth."

Representative Ayanna Pressley (an American politician) – Congresswoman describes her experience with hair loss, "I am making my peace with Alopecia", she said. The revelation-filled year in regard to her hair loss seems to have begun in 2020. The lawmaker created a vulnerable, frank, revealing, and emotionally moving video.

Prior to her hair loss, Pressley was well-known for her braids, which served as an inspiration to many young girls. In a deeply personal video, courtesy of the Root, she said, "I am ready now because I want to be freed." Baring all to the camera, she confessed "I didn't have the luxury of mourning what felt like the loss of a limb". The feisty freshman congresswoman who was known for her trademark Senegalese twists and braids felt the need to explain to the young girls who took pride in her natural hairstyles and had never seen braided hair on such a famous politician. Now that she is starting to embrace her new life, she is brave by starting a dialogue about Alopecia.

Selma Blair (an American actress) – If Selma Blair is someone you follow online, you are likely also following her public journey with Multiple Sclerosis (MS). The actress has always been as open with her fans about her health issues, her hair loss is no different.

In a moment from the actress's newest documentary, "Introducing, Selma Blair," her son, who was 7 years old at the time, cuts off his mother's hair before she had a life-altering stem cell transplant in 2019. Blair has repeatedly stood confidently for pictures while sporting no hair.

Sara Sampaio (a Portuguese model) – The fashion icon and Victoria's Secret model is living with Trichotillomania. She acknowledged that avoiding touching her brows is the key to having "fuller" brows in an Instagram (IG) Question & Answer session. Sampaio pulls on her hair a lot because of her Trichotillomania, which has left her with several bald and thinning spots that she has to fill in. Sampaio is undoubtedly not alone; more than 10 million people in the United States alone suffer from Trichotillomania.

Jada Pinkett-Smith (an American actress and talk show host) – The celebrity first discussed her battle with alopecia on a 2018 episode of her Facebook Watch show, "Red Table Talk." "It was terrifying when it first started," said Jada. "I was in the shower one day and I just had handfuls of hair in my hands and I was just like, oh my god, am I going bald?" She gets her inspiration from this and keeps cutting her hair short.

July 2021, the "Girls Trip" actress, posted a video on social media of her brand-new buzz cut. In the selfie-style clip, she moved and modeled her head to give her viewers a good look. She explained that her new look was inspired by her daughter. "Willow made me do it because it was time to let go BUT ... my 50s are about to be Divinely lit with this shed (emojis)." One fan said, "Welcome to the bald squad.."

Kristin Davis (an American actress) – Every 'Sex and the City episode feature Kristin Davis' thick hair, which is impossible to overlook. Nevertheless, Davis began to see her strands thinning nearly right away after the fan-favorite show's filming finally wrapped up. Simply put, "My hair just was not what it used to be. It was very fine, like it had gone away; there just was hardly any hair there," she said.

The actress first ignored her thinning hair but eventually recognized she needed a remedy. "It's always been not quite that easy, but because I had a lot of hair, the professionals could help me make it look nice," Davis said. "It's not like I woke up and I had Charlotte hair."

Alyssa Milano (an American actress) – Star of "Who's the Boss?" and "Charmed", Alyssa Milano has been outspoken about the trauma her body underwent after developing COVID-19, which led to her hair loss. She posted a video on Instagram in which she discussed her experience.

"Thought I'd show you what COVID-19 does to your hair. Please take this seriously," Milano wrote in the caption as she brushed her hair as strands of hair fell from her head. "One brushing, this is my hair loss,"

Viola Davis (an American actress) – In an interview, Academy Award winner, Viola Davis previously described having alopecia at the age of 28. "I woke up one day, and it looked like I had a Mohawk. Big splash of bald on the top of my head", the actress said. Davis felt embarrassed by the abrupt loss of her hair. "I am telling you, I have spent so much of my life not feeling comfortable in my skin. I am just so not there anymore." She gave an explanation, having never exposed her natural hair for years, hiding behind wigs. "It was a crutch, not an enhancement", she claimed. "I was so desperate for people to think that I was beautiful. I had to be liberated from that feeling to a certain extent."

Just Imagine It

If you were bald, how would you look? This is a common question that many people ask, so if you've ever asked it of yourself, you're not alone. Many people have surely wondered what some of our favorite celebrities would look like without hair, as we continue to dig at why people are so curious about celebrities.

The following images were produced, or "Balderized", and are easily accessible online thanks to BalderaZZi.com. There are currently many smartphone apps and simple PhotoShop adjustments that may be done to get a hairless look.

* * *

"Balderized" Celebrities

After viewing the photos of some of the most beautiful and famous people on the planet, again, I suggest asking yourself, if seeing your favorite celebrity with hair loss changes your perception of them. If given the opportunity, I would ask them, "How do you perceive yourself after seeing yourself with a completely bald head?"

Several apps will easily display an unaltered image of your face modified to how you would look if you had a bald head. That is if you are curious to learn how a bald head might modify your overall appearance or self-perception.

Depending on whether or not you have impending hair loss, this can be a very sobering remedy; nevertheless, for many, it might just be the solution to a burning "What if?" issue. The visual will leave no room for doubt, there it is, staring right back at you. Although many of the apps seem to be developed for men, like many other things, I think the application can be very useful to women. So much so, I used it to answer a few burning questions I had of my own.

Check out Chapter Eleven (11) for the social experiment and surveys.

* * *

Overwhelming Thoughts

Recently, I sent out an invitation to some of my hair loss clients to share a few instances that made them uncomfortable. Their experiences vary from random encounters to scheduled appointments, everyday life, etc.

Jennifer K.

 • I don't like for people to get up close, are they wondering, if this is not my hair?

- A few weeks ago, a man that I know only in the context of the church, made a comment about me wearing a wig.

Sandra F.

- When getting my yearly dental cleaning, do my dentist and his hygienist see that my hair is not real?

- I'm now a widow; in an argument, my deceased husband made a comment about my baldness.

- My primary care doctor, when she places the otoscope in my ears, can she see my bald spots?

Eliza S.

- I'm dating now, will I be desirable to others?

- I was given a compliment about my hair, and she then whispered to me "I know that is not your real hair."

Sissy P.

- Is that yours (referring to my wig)?

- I hate to look at my hair (without my wig on).

- When I'm deceased, will everyone see my secret!?

Many people constantly hear a critical inner voice nagging at them. This critical internal conversation frequently demeans them and dwells on life's imperfections. Therefore, it can be challenging for people to advance if they haven't already silenced their critical inner voice.

Shhh-ing the Inner Voice

Have you had similar concerns, thoughts, or feelings? How would you like to end this self-defeating internal conversation after reading these shared experiences of my clients'? The next time the effort is made to venture beyond your comfort zone, your inner voice that says "you can't" becomes much louder and renders you even more vulnerable. You need to break this loop. First, by responding to the questions below, define the characteristics of the negative internal discourse. Knowing the characteristics of the negative mental chatter will make it easier to silence.

Who is Criticizing You?

- From where does the voice appear to be coming?

- What is the voice's volume?

- Does the voice repeat itself constantly?

- Is the voice speaking slowly or quickly?

- What tone does the voice have?

You can silence the voice now that you are more cognizant of it than you were before. Make a conscious decision to alter the voice's characteristics to achieve this. You accomplish this by visualizing the same voice with different vocal characteristics.

What happens if you visualize a volume dial and lower the negative internal voice's volume? What happens when the internal voice of negativity is turned up? Find what prevents the negative internal voice from having an impact on you. The likelihood is that the voice will have less impact the quieter it is. Once you figure it out, it's actually very easy. This method's fundamental premise is to actively control your thoughts rather than letting them flow randomly. Here, you are actively choosing how you want to hear your inner voice.

What happens when the voice is sped up so quickly that it is almost unintelligible? What happens if you slooooooow the voice down 'til it is deep and distorted? You will feel so much better whenever you have greater control over your inner dialogue; the negative internal dialogue will have a decreasingly negative effect on you.

Pump Up the Volume

The positive internal dialogue will undergo the same treatment as the negative internal dialogue but in reverse. The effects of the internal dialogue can be amplified by doing a variety of things to support it.

Take a moment to silently thank yourself whenever you hear yourself saying something encouraging and uplifting. Reinforce the action as you start to speak positively to yourself in your thoughts. You will find yourself seeing yourself in the way you want to more frequently if you reward yourself for doing so.

Give yourself permission to hear that inner voice of positivity. Allow it to permeate every area of your body. Every time you hear that brilliant, uplifting voice inside of you, shout it out as loudly as you can as if it were coming from the biggest audio speakers you've ever heard. You will experience the vibrations of positivity coursing throughout your entire body, more when the volume is turned up. So, pump up the volume when you want to really experience it!

Even if you hear your positive inner voice more frequently, it occasionally will disguise an uplifting thought as a question. "Am I beautiful?", for instance. Although the tone may be one like a question, the sentence is actually a declaration. By transforming the phrase, "I am beautiful", into a statement, you can increase the strength of your inner voice. Try it out by mentally repeating it a few times. Then change the sentence into an exclamation by saying, "I am beautiful!", to amplify your inner voice even more. When you mentally repeat it several times, pay attention to how you feel about it. Declare this loudly in your head! You'll shout out the doubt, therefore believing in yourself.

The core concept is to start trusting yourself in the same way that the world's most successful people trust their internal voices and believe in themselves.

Others might try to impose their own inadequacies and limitations onto you. Any unintentional negativity by friends, family, and coworkers can be avoided by saying the following words: "Abort, abort, abort." If you find someone offering you a negative opinion, terrible advice, or putting their restrictions inside of you, privately say the words "abort, abort". That one powerful word, "abort", will act as a reminder to you to destroy any negative thoughts that may have entered your mind.

Breaking through the B.S.

Earlier, I posed the question, "Is self-esteem just a 'Belief System'?" It is very probable, before you could answer for yourself, my exclamatory response was, "YES! It undoubtedly is!" This section of the book is where we put everything into action.

If you are dealing with low self-esteem, lack of confidence, depression, emotional issues, and insecurities because of your hair loss, I am going to share ways to break the B.S. (Belief Systems) affecting you negatively and how to adopt new ones!

Building Confidence

The relevance – the necessity – of understanding how crucial self-acceptance is as a component of the process of addressing and overcoming poor self-belief is often overlooked in most of the literature and information on self- esteem and confidence building.

The adage "A house built on sand shall not stand" perfectly captures the relevance and significance of self-acceptance in successful self-esteem and confidence building. In this case, it means that you're much more likely to succeed in developing a positive and lasting self-belief and self-image; only after you've undergone a rigorously honest self-evaluation of who and where you really are in life at the present time. You may effectively begin to construct your self-esteem and a new positive self-image on the psychological foundation created by this honest self-evaluation and acceptance of yourself as you are, hair loss and all.

Without it, any program for boosting self-esteem and confidence is doomed to failure. As long as you continue to deny the reality of certain aspects of your personality and/ or appearance that you find objectionable, or refuse to accept, this denial and/or nonacceptance will act as a mental barrier, preventing your continued development and growth.

This is not meant to suggest that you should try to make yourself "like" the aspects of yourself that you dislike; rather, it is meant to emphasize the importance of realizing that the aspects of yourself that you find to be unflattering will only continue to be so as long as you attempt to mentally battle them, avoid them, or, in other words, refuse to accept them as a part of who you are.

You can start the process of eradicating these items' ability to undermine your self-belief and self-image by learning to absorb and accept them, not "liking" them but accepting them nonetheless.

Mirror Exercise

The use of a full-length mirror is part of an activity that is well known to be successful in promoting self-acceptance. That is especially beneficial for those whose self-esteem and confidence have been badly influenced by some aspect of their physical appearance. If you have one or are able to obtain one, set aside some private time to stand in front of it fully undressed; without the aid of any soft or complementary lighting, cosmetics, or other accessories.

Make a mental note of the emotions and ideas that come to mind as you look over your head, face, and body; especially when you consider your hair loss. If you are like most people, you will discover that some features or areas of yourself are more difficult to examine than others. This is common and doesn't necessarily have anything to do with overall self-confidence as such. Some people live with some element or aspect of themselves, particularly their physical selves, that they just do not like and have felt unable to accept. As a result, the "thing" ends up acquiring such negative power and depth in their minds that it seriously harms their self-esteem and confidence.

Case in point, we are focusing on hair loss; however, it could also have to do with being overweight or underweight, showing signs of aging, physical damage of some kind, or any other of the various "defects" that you observe. Being in touch with the feelings that these things elicit is challenging; the initial inclination is to turn away from, deny, or refuse to embrace whatever it is that you find upsetting.

Start this exercise, by keeping in mind that its goal is not to make you enjoy everything about yourself; rather, it's to help you accept yourself entirely for who and what you are, including what you like and do not like.

Inhale, exhale, breathe deeply and make an effort to direct your attention toward the part of yourself that is causing you the most stress. If you are unable to tackle it this time, promise yourself that you will do so tomorrow and then follow through on that promise. The following day, repeat the mirror practice and make an extra effort to concentrate on the part or location that is causing you the most pain.

Creating Empowerment

Your thoughts and beliefs determine whether you lead a happy life or a miserable one. A change in beliefs is the foundation of all development. Therefore, the first thing you need to know is that ANY belief may be changed. Bernie Siegel, a well-known physician, and spiritual guide is well renowned for his reports of fascinating findings from research on multiple personality disorders.

According to the personality the patient was displaying at the time, measurable changes in body chemistry, physical characteristics, and illnesses like diabetes would develop and disappear in these tests and many others. The fact that the patients' thoughts and beliefs about who they were at the time, truly changed their body systems. Think about the effects your beliefs have on you. So, what is a belief really, anyway? Ultimately, they are ideas or thoughts that are supported by references. Imagine the thought being a table and the evidence, or references, that support it being the legs. The key to changing a belief is to knock the legs out from under it. And, how do we do that? We create doubt.

Consider this: were there not things you once believed and possibly would have defended vehemently, but today you'd be ashamed to acknowledge? What occurred then, that caused you to doubt? Evidence. There were enough instances that contradicted your beliefs for you to begin to doubt them. You challenged it. And if you doubt something long enough, you'll start to doubt everything.

Building proof for your new beliefs also is necessary if you wish to modify a belief. Begin to consider your outdated, undesirable thinking. Question the source of the information and its reliability. Determine who told you and your level of certainty regarding their accuracy. If there is any evidence that contradicts your beliefs, ask yourself if you have seen it.

Consider how you would cross-examine your beliefs as a lawyer. Do you have evidence to support its truth beyond a reasonable doubt? In that case, give up on the idea because it has no basis.

Seek evidence that the beliefs you desire are true. What instances do you notice that demonstrate the viability of your desires, even though up until this point you didn't think they were possible? TAKE ACTION because every action you take to achieve your goals, regardless of whether you think it is attainable, increases your confidence level and your capability to believe in them.

You are choosing the beliefs that will empower you because you are reading this book. As a life coach, I understand the importance of improving well-being and strengthening mental fitness. I cannot stress enough, you are not alone.

Don't Ask, Don't Tell

"Stephanie, I felt like a spotlight was shining directly on me", my client cried. I reached my left hand over towards the box of Kleenex on my desk and handed her a few. Between sniffles, Jacquie begins to relive the moment as she begins to describe her experience.

Just a couple of days after her last appointment with me, she went to the mall to pick up a few items to accessorize a new outfit she had just bought. "I was really feeling good about myself that day. You had recently done my hair, my makeup was on point, and I had just received a notice of a speaking engagement that I landed", she exclaimed! "I was on cloud nine and felt on top of the world". It was then that I was soon to learn that a chance meeting with a complete stranger changed the trajectory of her day and ultimately how she saw herself.

It was a similar story that I had heard before. Has this happened to you like my client? Or were you the complete stranger? Long story short, the women, while shopping, exchanged niceties. The stranger, admiring her hair, asked if that was my client's hair because it was so beautiful. My client went off "script" and didn't retort "Yes" as I have always advised all my clients. My rationale is anything you buy, "it's yours", right? I know what the stranger meant, and I also know what the impact of that line of questioning felt like for my client.

Every positive feeling she felt prior to this encounter was quickly and crudely erased. Jacquie said, "Stephanie, I was at a loss for words. I began to think," she continued, "if I told her it was a wig, would I have to explain my diagnosis of Alopecia?" I could hear how dejected my client was. Ultimately, she told the woman, "Yes, it is." However, not for the reason I suggested. She was ashamed. This complete stranger gave her a glance that Jacquie was unsure of. Did she believe her, or not? This uncertainty additionally led to her uneasiness and self-consciousness. She felt like a liar, she felt insecure and she felt like she wanted to go home. My client left the mall without purchasing anything.

I listened, as I knew, the importance of finding out what she was feeling that very moment. She needed reassurance that someone was listening and understood her. That was the only way for her to overcome and deal with this. As I provided her service during her appointment, I asked a few "how" and "why" questions. I first needed to gauge her feelings. It was painfully obvious the level of hurt she felt, even as she recounted the experience. As much as I would like to say otherwise, it was emotional for me as well; regardless of how many of my clients are subjected to similar intrusions in their lives. I will never be OK with it. These intrusions, whether by family, friends, co-workers, or perfect strangers are unacceptable. Regardless of the intent, harmless or not.

This dichotomy even exists with people who do not experience hair loss. I have clients with beautiful and full naturally growing hair. They too have encountered people who give these "reluctant" compliments or toxic praise. Simply meaning, the hair is beautiful and downright gorgeous and warrants being addressed.

Women love compliments, especially about their hair. However, this is prevalent in modern life, although we do not always see it. The term "toxic praise" refers to the use of praise for manipulative purposes, i.e., to either mute or promote particular results, feelings, and/or sentiments in other people in order to achieve a desired effect. This may be, but need not be, the result of the praise-giver having a conscious desire or awareness to be manipulative.

I have had clients and witnessed videos on social media of women taking time to actually part, comb, or section through their hair in order to prove it is their own naturally, growing hair.

It is ridiculous! It elicits negative emotions in people without hair loss to have this happen to them. Can you imagine how those with hair loss feel?

Are people truly asking because it looks so good that it could not possibly be real? I don't know. However, I do have a suggestion. Don't ask, don't tell. If you see someone with a gorgeous mane and beautiful hairstyle and would like to ask them a question, by all means, do. Simply, tell them how much you love their hair and ask who their hairstylist is. That is the safest way to go without being offensive.

* * *

Thank you for making me so wonderfully complex! Your workmanship is marvelous—how well I know it. *Psalms 139:14 (NLT)*

CHAPTER 6

MOURNING THE LOSS

An Emotional Toll

❝ Ma'am...I am losing my hair. I need help, not sympathy", she said to me. During a consultation, a prospective client expressed her mounting frustration in getting help for her sudden hair loss. It's unfortunate that her personal hurt and pain wouldn't allow her to accept the help I was prepared to extend to her. She came into the consultation armed with a defensive attitude. She was in pain. I understood her and didn't take it personally. I do not think she truly believed anyone could help her, but felt an obligation to come to the appointment her best friend had scheduled with me on her behalf.

Hair loss can take an overwhelming emotional toll on people. As a professional specializing in this field, I quickly learned that people can and most likely will mourn the loss of their hair. Similar to the death of a dearly departed family member or friend.

Loss is a significant element of life that necessitates an investment in oneself. People may require assistance in dealing with loss, anxiety, and despair. Emotions that, if not resolved, accumulate and intensify over time. They may struggle to cope with life's daily stressors, such as work, relationships, or finances, and must be taught skills and tactics to make stress more manageable. If individuals are unable to participate in social events, activities, interests, or pleasures due to anxiety, they require tools to retrain the brain to turn off anxiety. If a loss has left them feeling empty, despondent, lonely, or alone, they may require assistance in finding ways to fill the vacuum. Many people are just getting by and need a new perspective to help them live a more fulfilling life.

Meet Them Where They Are

"Meet them where they are" is a popular expression these days. But what exactly does it mean? What effect does it have on our personal and professional interactions with others? We should endeavor to connect with individuals in a way that is effective for them, regardless of whom we are working with. It's a difficult lesson to learn if you're on a road that entails wanting to help others. Sometimes you want the other person to heal, to grow, to learn, to advance, more than they do. Teachers witness it with their pupils, physicians witness it with their patients, parents witness it with their children, and friends witness it with their friends.

If we are truly in the business of helping others, we must learn to meet them where they are. As a Hair Replacement Specialist, I had to learn this; and as a coach and transformation consultant, I still have to remind myself of it. People are not always willing to accept assistance. Some people are content to take one or two baby steps, whilst others are eager to jump in with both feet.

Is it Sympathy or Empathy?

Empathy isn't the same as sympathy. Whereas sympathy is defined as "feeling for someone," empathy is defined as "feeling as someone." For example, you may feel horrible for your client, or more accurately, you may feel bad about their circumstance. Many individuals define empathy as "placing yourself in their shoes" and feeling as they would.

We should practice listening with empathy. Listening empathetically requires the ability to set oneself aside. Listening without judgment is required, even if you hold an opposing viewpoint or disagree with your client. It distinguishes between acknowledging, approving, and agreeing. Your point of view is immaterial. You are not attempting to address their problem. You are simply paying attention and tuning in to how they are feeling. Does that seem contradictory? That is not the case. And this is where many people get it wrong when it comes to empathy and putting themselves in the shoes of others. Putting oneself aside also means not considering how you would feel if it were your situation. Consider how that would relate to your interactions with someone who is suffering from losing their hair.

The Golden Rule: Is it that Simple?

Like most, I am sure you are familiar with The Golden Rule: Do unto others as you would have them do unto you. Most people interpret this to mean deciding how you want others to treat you, and then treating them accordingly. If you're talking about respect or being nice, that seems straightforward enough. However, the simple scenario of someone becoming ill clearly demonstrates the flaw in this understanding of the golden rule. Do you like being pampered and having someone look after you when you're sick? Or would you rather be left alone in your solitude? If you prefer doting, you could dote on people who are sick while adhering to the golden rule. But what if they'd rather be alone? You are treating them as you would like to be treated. But that is not what they desire. They wish to be alone. So, here's the real meaning of the golden rule:

The Golden Rule: Determine what others would like done to them and then do it. It is not what you'd like to have done for yourself.

Now, let's look at "empathy means placing yourself in another person's shoes". Many people get stuck because they envision themselves in the other person's shoes, asking themselves, "How would I feel if it were me?" However, by doing so, they are putting themselves in the predicament. It's a step closer to empathy, but if they look down, they'll notice they're still wearing their own shoes, not the other person's.

Putting it in Practice

To fully empathize, you must adopt your client's viewpoint rather than your own. Rather than view what your client is saying or experiencing through your own filters—your own experiences, beliefs, and feelings—your goal is to remain open and see them from their point of view.

- Do I feel sorry for my client? If that's the case, it's sympathy.

- Is it possible that I'm talking too much or comparing their predicament to something in my own life? If this is the case, it is not a negative thing. However, it would be preferable if you were aware of this and returned your attention to your client. Refrain from talking about oneself in order to discover common ground. First, just listen and concentrate on them, not on yourself.

- Is it possible that I'm seeing myself in their shoes? If so, great. Now go one step further and see if you still have your own shoes on. Remove all judgmental thoughts, such as "this is bad". Instead of thinking, "If this were me, I would feel _____," consider, "If I were them, how would I feel, knowing what I know about them?" Ask more questions if you don't know enough about them, and their situation, to tell the difference between how they may be feeling and how they would feel.

The key takeaway is simply because you experience emotion in response to what your client is saying, it does not imply that you are empathizing. It is critical to practice limiting this and to be aware that you are experiencing your own emotions, not those of others. You must first stop experiencing your own emotions in order to pick up on someone else's. Then, you can pick up on another person's feelings by experiencing their energetic field and studying physical signs such as tears, tone of voice, posture, language, and expression. Then you may envision what it would be like from their point of view as if you were them. Your empathy in this situation isn't based on a gut instinct, but rather on thorough observation and carefully assuming their position.

Bottom line, no one wants you to feel sorry for them, or sympathy. Practice making them feel understood, affirmed, validated, and that they can trust you.

Simple Change of Scenery

Ms. Gossett requested a consultation as she was continually losing hair and didn't know why. She was very specific about the general time she wanted to see me, "I need your earliest appointment or your latest appointment". Though I try very hard to accommodate requests, I have specific times in which I schedule my consultations throughout my work days. However, we were able to secure a date and time that worked perfectly for us both.

The day and time of her appointment came, and she was an utter delight. A mature woman, small business owner, wife, and mother...very proud San Antonian. The one thing that she was not proud of understandably, was her hair loss. As we discussed her options and the services I could provide to her, she told me a little about her previous hairstylist and how I was referred to her.

Her previous relationship with her stylist was for 9+ years, she hated the thought of leaving her. Well, I understand firsthand the relationship that can be developed over time between hair professionals and clients. It can be special and long-lasting. The treatment plan that I developed for her could easily be administered at my facility; she could still receive the cosmetic services she loved through her stylist. I let her know how we could coordinate that and offered she could share my contact information with her stylist if she had any questions for me. Ms. Gossett, for a fleeting moment, seemed excited about the prospect of that happening. Until she looked at me and asked, "Do you remember me requesting your 'earliest appointment or your latest appointment' when I called you earlier?" Yes, of course, I did. I nodded my head in affirmation.

That is the same request she had made for the last 18 months to her former stylist. She wanted to be the first client seen in the morning or the last client seen in the evening. It wasn't because she was a difficult woman, a prima donna, or similar temperament. As her hair loss advanced, she required special styling techniques that were embarrassing to her. Her prior stylist, whom she was fond of, worked in an open-floor salon where there was little to no privacy. Even when she was accommodated as being the first or the last, there was always someone else there, watching and she felt so insecure. She mentioned it to her stylist, but her stylist did not seem to understand or was just limited to the space in which she could provide services to her. To top it off, it was a dual-licensed facility; there were barbers and cosmetologists also employed there. Not only were there other women she felt were able to see her balding scalp, but men as well. She was mortified. All she was asking for was a change of scenery, a private area, or another room.

I personally believe, as professionals, we have the duty to provide respect and empathy to our clients at all times. As a professional cosmetologist in the state of Texas, our governing body, the Texas Department of Licensing and Regulation (TDLR), has a platform for human trafficking. All licensed beauty professionals in our area are mandated reporters. Yet, some don't have the courtesy of providing privacy to those who need and crave it. There are general cosmetology practitioners that only provide styling services; they do not offer specialized care, treatment, or services for those losing their hair. You can't call yourself a hair loss professional if you don't have the basic requirements for privacy. Never share the details of another client's hair loss issue....and you won't have to if they come to you with a completely obvious bald head for everyone's viewing. Someone discreet, secretive, and self-conscious about the state of their hair underneath the wig, system, unit, sew-in, etc. never divulge their secret.

Providing a specialized service or space sometimes is not appreciated by everyone. However, for those clients who need it, it can be life-changing for them. I provide closed-door services to my clients who require and prefer "privacy". As The Hair Replacement Coach, I emphasize to all my students the need for closed-door services once you begin servicing clients in that special demographic and that level of care.

I attempted to explain to the client the difference between a cosmetologist/hairstylist and a hair loss specialist like myself. I did not think it was by any malicious intent that her stylist would not comply with her need. She did address her want (wanting specific times for an appointment), beautiful hair services, and a great relationship; however, her stylist was unable to satisfy her need for privacy because she did not have spacing for an office area, partition, or other means of seclusion. It is similar to attempting to solve "the XY".

* * *

Fear thou not; for I am with thee: be not dismayed; for I am thy God: I will strengthen thee; yea, I will help thee; yea, I will uphold thee with the right hand of my righteousness. *Isaiah 41:10 (KJV)*

CHAPTER 7
MIND AND BODY CONNECTION

Undisputed Fact

I t's practically an undisputed fact that a woman losing her hair may suffer from low self-image, lack of self-esteem, and no self-confidence in certain situations. Not only is there an internal voice recorder influencing her on how she feels about and sees herself; but there may also be external factors as well. Laughter, stares, and unwelcomed comments from strangers, along with negative remarks from family, friends, co-workers, and in-laws (and outlaws), whether intentionally well-meaning or not, can catapult one into spiraling down the rabbit hole.

At the time I began writing this book, the importance of studying self-image had long since been acknowledged. It has been extensively covered in literature. This is due to the fact that the practice of self-image is useful, efficient, and has astonishingly effective results.

I began making a few observations of clients and how they related to their self-image challenges. This began my journey of understanding the emotional components of how losing your hair can affect people. It opened a new world for me of many theories and practices of motivation, personal development, and self-help from many of the great thinkers like Iyanla Vanzant, Lisa Nichols, Maxwell Maltz, Tony Robbins, Zig Ziglar, and others. My appetite to learn more about this phenomenon cultivated an intense desire for more. I became a voracious reader and devoured books by reading one after the other. This led me to study, take multiple tests, and ultimately become certified as a Personal Life Coach. These books and training confirmed and changed my life as I began recounting my experiences with clients and how they related to their self-image challenges.

Are you familiar with the quote by Helen Exley, "Books can be dangerous. The best ones should be labeled 'This could change your life.'"? There are many books that I have read that changed my life. I pray that I do not sound arrogant or self-absorbed. I do sincerely hope that my deliberate attempt to share what I have learned and those experiences shared within these writings does for you what other books have done for me.

Self-image Discovery

A large number of the apparent experiences I had noticed with my clients are explained by self-image discovery. It is the shared denominator—the driving force for a lot of their thoughts, both positive and negative. The key is having a solid and realistic self-image that you can live with in order to truly "live" a true and authentic life, which is to find life relatively enjoyable. You need to be acceptable to "you." You must possess a sound sense of self-worth. You need to be able to trust and believe in yourself. You need to be able to express yourself effectively without feeling like you have to hide who you are. To function well in the real world, you need to have a self that is true to reality. You must be honest with yourself about both your abilities and limitations and have a thorough understanding of who you are. Your self-image must be an accurate representation of "you", not more or less than who you are.

Doubt, in my opinion, is the first thing that women experience when they begin to acknowledge that they are experiencing hair loss. As women, we are extremely attached to our hair. When losing it, they want to know whether they are still attractive without it. Women have a preconceived notion of who they are, and it takes them some time to realize who they are now when that image of them is gone.

Solving the XY

Similar to Dr. Maxwell Maltz, who observed that many of his plastic surgery patients had expectations that were not met by the procedures he performed on them, I have also found similar outcomes from my experience with some clients and the services I offer. A surgical cosmetic service and a non-surgical hair replacement service can be distinguished from one another on the surface. One is simply permanent, whereas the other is not.

There are, however, advantages and disadvantages to each, as well as justifications for choosing one over the other. Despite the similarities in our respective professional goals, Dr. Maltz and I both strive to assist our patients and/or clients to feel their best after receiving services. Years ago, he sought a way to assist his patients in setting the aim of a successful outcome by envisioning that successful outcome. The XY problem is illustrated by patients who believe surgery will address their issues. Thinking about your attempted solution rather than your actual problem is a way to understand the logic behind an XY problem.

In other words, you are trying to solve problem X and believe that method Y would work, but when you run into problems, you ask about Y rather than X. Maltz started wondering about, for instance, whether setting goals is effective. He discovered that the connection between the mind and the body is how self-affirmation and mental visualization techniques work. In order to create a positive outer objective, he provided ways for creating a positive inner objective. His strategy depends on this focus on inner attitudes since he argues that an individual can never achieve greater success than what they envision for themselves inwardly.

I Want That

She was a new potential client and scheduled a consultation with me from a referral. I gathered basic information during the telephone call to access what type of consultation she needed. She was looking for a specific wig and look. While securing her contact information and confirming the date and time of our meeting, I asked her to bring me an "inspiration photo" to the consultation appointment. An "inspiration photo" is a tool I use to assess client expectations. It allows me to see the look they want, while also giving me the opportunity to determine if this look is something that can, or even should, be attempted.

Clients typically enter my facility with at least one of two emotions: excitement or nervousness. Hey, perhaps it combines elements of both. They are undoubtedly really eager to receive whatever service or therapy is coming; but as they try something new, their worries start to surface.

As a specialist in hair loss, I am quite accustomed to this and try to make them feel at ease. After all, our shared objective is to help people feel and look their best. It's also normal if their anxiety causes me to feel hesitant and question if they will accept my complete honesty if I offer my professional assessment of the new look or service they are requesting.

Establishing reasonable expectations with the client is one method I enlist to help us both feel at ease and confident about the choice. Encouraging them and staying positive, I am always truthful about what I think will happen in the end.

If a customer brings in a photo of a famous person, an Instagram influencer, a model, etc. to demonstrate the type of wig style, haircut, or color they desire, we have a discussion about it. Especially if their hair type differs significantly from that of the particular A-lister. Hair type is less important if they want a wig fitted and styled compared to whether or not their facial shape will emphasize the look they want. This makes it easier for them to decide whether or not they want to pursue it; I am more likely to have a satisfied customer at the conclusion of the visit.

However, that is not always the case as in the consultation above. When this client came in, it was evident Cleo was a calm, introverted, gentle, and unassuming soul. Her voice was very quiet, so I had to listen very attentively to the answers from the questions I asked her about herself and what I could do for her. She said, "I want that". When she showed me the "inspiration photo" of the wig style she desired, it was totally different from what I'd imagined for her. It was a beautiful trendy pixie-cut style and the model who wore it was simply gorgeous. Although I didn't imagine that Ms. Cleo would pick this style of wig, I honestly thought she could rock it. Her skin was flawless, her face and bone structure would easily pull this look off. She just had to know she could rock it to pull it off. Something I was unsure of.

Nonetheless, after visiting with her and agreeing to transform her into this new look, I cut, curled, and styled this cute pixie-cut wig for her. I fit it to her head and performed precise finishing touches as I turned her around smiling, admiring my work. Her first reaction to seeing herself in the hand mirror perplexed me.

I wanted to know what she thought of her new hairstyle. "The hair is beautiful; you did a great job. It doesn't look like a wig, at all!" Cleo exclaimed, as she touched the hair in a trance, and ran her fingers through it. "I don't look like her." I wondered, who was "her" she was trying to look like... the model? Immediately, she came to herself and said, that she loved it but her eyes could not hide her feelings. I asked if she was sure, and she reassured me that she loved the wig and the style. What I noticed was, her self-image did not align with what she aspired to be.

Even as diligent as I had been in an attempt to gauge her expectations, she still was disappointed. Had I felt that the wig's look wasn't a fit for her, I would have recommended something else. Contrary to Cleo, I have encountered previous clients who initially struck me as having a quiet, shy demeanor; however, when they tried on a wig, they embraced and owned that persona of the wig. That's why I have many of my clients name their wigs. They may at times take on the personality of those wigs and the feelings they evoke.

Cleo's self-imposed image of herself would not allow her to see what I saw in her. I saw a beautiful, striking woman who could have easily pulled off that look and many others. That is something I cannot say of everyone. However, how quiet, calm, and gentle of a personality, I saw into the depths of who she was and had the potential to be. After all, she brought the picture to me. She on some level aspired to be, do, look, and feel something different. In the end, she didn't believe she could.

That result happens less than it does often. However, when there's a deeper, emotional issue involved, regardless of my efforts during the consultation to discuss options, nothing is guaranteed. This might take a little longer than expected for my client's appointment, but it most often means the difference between a happily ever after and a less-than-ideal finish.

* * *

Each time he said, "My grace is all you need. My power works best in weakness." So now I am glad to boast about my weaknesses, so that the power of Christ can work through me. *2 Corinthians 12:9 (NLT)*

CHAPTER 8
PROFESSIONAL IMPACT

Beyond the Roots of Hair

A hair replacement specialist does more than just change a woman's appearance by applying a wig. She changes a woman's inner self.

The attachment she forms is temporary. However, it may actually alter the psyche. I decided a long time ago that this is a huge responsibility, and that I owe it to both my clients and myself to understand what I'm doing. Without specific knowledge and training, no reputable hair loss professional would attempt to provide this specialized care. So, since changing a woman's appearance has the capability of changing her inner woman, I always believed it was my obligation to gain specialized expertise in that subject as well.

There are published compilations of case histories in which cosmetic surgery, particularly facial plastic surgery, has given many patients a new lease on life. Similarly, Non-Surgical Hair Replacement (NSHR) can produce similar results for individuals who use it. There are accounts of astonishing changes in an individual's personality that occur rather rapidly and drastically when their face is changed. I was overjoyed with my results in this regard, especially when it came to the changes I saw in my clients after experiencing my non-surgical attachments of wigs and hair prostheses. However, like many others before me, I learned more from my mistakes than from my accomplishments. Some clients' personalities did not change as a result of their attachment services. In most cases, a person with moderate to severe hair loss or some "scarring" of the scalp, who had no prospect of hair growth enhanced by an NSHR attachment service, saw an almost instantaneous increase in self-esteem and self-confidence. However, in some instances, the client continued to feel insecure and inadequate. In short, these clients felt, acted, and behaved as if they still had no hair on their heads at all.

This revealed to me that changing one's physical appearance was not "the" true path to changing one's personality. Something else was occasionally altered by hair replacement, but not always. When this "something else" was rebuilt, the person transformed. When this "something else" was not reconstructed, the person remained the same, even though her physical attributes were greatly changed.

Hair Stylists and Bartenders

I hesitated a little bit before I started writing a book about this topic. For some readers, any book I would write on the subject may appear a little out of the ordinary for a hair loss specialist to publish a book containing some simple points of psychology. Going outside of the "stringent system" of the "ideology of psychology" and looking for explanations about human behavior in the disciplines of physics and anatomy, in relation to the emotional component of hair loss, may be seen by some as even more unconventional. My response is that whether she would have it that way or not, any competent expert on hair loss is, and must be, a therapist.

Consider the fact that both professions, bartenders and hairstylists, are unofficial therapists. Always have been, always will be. Therefore, bartenders and hairstylists are fortunate to be the people who get to engage with clients and be present in their life at extremely vulnerable periods, whether you are pouring wine or hair color. We become experts in more topics and subjects than you can think of, thanks to our experiences and the knowledge we learn. We are familiar with you, we adore you, and as a bonus, we also get paid by you.

COVID-19 Sheltering in Place

In 2020, during the coronavirus pandemic, the fundamentals of a "shelter-in-place" order were pretty obvious: remain at home. Nevertheless, there were many "important" activity exemptions in that order. Additionally, it was far from a situation where you would seek shelter during a serious emergency, such as a tornado or an active shooting. Millions of Americans eventually became familiar with the specifics of the shelter-in-place order and its numerous caveats for "vital" activities as towns, states, and the federal government took increasingly strong action to limit the spread of the new coronavirus. It was a new, uncomfortable, and scary time for us all.

To restrict the transmission of the virus, such an order is meant to compel social segregation, or to keep people apart from one another. Going outside does not pose any inherent risks. Being near other infected people, whether they realize it or not, is dangerous.

Essential Businesses

I never could have imagined the potential impact of COVID-19. I am unsure if initially, many of us truly knew, what was ahead of us. It wasn't until only essential businesses were allowed to open. I'll never forget it, Tuesday, March 17, 2020, St. Patrick's Day, and it was the last time for thirteen (13) weeks that I would be able to open up my hair loss facility to clients. At that moment, I wasn't aware of it, that I was closing down after serving my last client for the day. I monitored the updates by San Antonio Mayor Ron Nirenberg, and Bexar County Judge Nelson Wolff; the rising numbers of those infected in the community, and the numerous calls by clients to cancel appointments. It wasn't until the following Monday, March 23, 2020, that the "Stay Home, Work Safe" emergency orders mandated citizens to stay at home; unless they had urgent tasks or essential work to do. On Tuesday at 11:59 p.m., the order went into effect. Unless it was extended, it was scheduled to last until April 9th. It would eventually be extended for weeks. And weeks. And more weeks.

However, with the mandated changes required by the Center for Disease Control (CDC) and Texas Department of Licensing & Regulation (TDLR) as a result of COVID-19, we felt that additional time was required for us to prepare for a safe return to work for us, as well as our clients. Not until June 22nd were we able to open the doors of Trinity Lace Wigs & Unisex Salon to our clients. There were several new protocols concerning safety, sanitation, and our business operations.

Impact of Sheltering-In

During our closure, I kept up with my clients via Zoom, phone calls, emails, and texts. I answered questions and made suggestions for some on what they could use, and how to perform some personal services to maintain their hair until our wig salon's reopening. For many clients, the thought of doing their own hair system was challenging for them. They were extremely happy to see me, as I was them, on their first visits back to my facility. There were others for whom the mere thought of having to personally service their own hair systems and wigs by themselves impacted them greatly. As I suspected, it would not be easy for them. However, as they recounted their personal experiences, I totally underestimated the emotional impact it had on them.

Nancy S

 I couldn't go shopping, I couldn't go to church, I couldn't get my hair done. Out of the many things I couldn't do during the COVID-19 shut down, I think one of the hardest was not being able to get my hair done. Ms. Stephanie has been taking care of me for about eleven (11) years now. I used to go to another hair replacement lady in the area, but she would at times forget to order my new wigs for my "change out" appointments. The quality of her service over time began to slip. When I heard about Ms. Stephanie, I made an appointment with her, tried her out, and never looked back.

I have scarring alopecia, and I've experienced about 80% of total hair loss on my head. I couldn't tell you what that looks like because it's been many years since I saw my head without a wig. I refuse to look in the mirror while I am getting serviced. Ms. Stephanie turns her styling chair away from the mirror as she removes my wig at each appointment. I never look into the mirror until my service is complete and my hair is on tight and right. It is my hair, I have the receipt, I own it. I identify with it. Intellectually I know that I have severe hair loss, but emotionally it is hard for me to look at it.

During the COVID-19 lockdown, I wanted to take care of my hair. I really did, but I could never take off my wig. I shampooed my hair while in the shower, and added tape when I felt it getting loose. I was scared to do too much to it because I didn't want to chance it coming off. For a few months, unable to get to my wig stylist, it was hard. Thank God, not many people actually saw me.

My job started working me remotely from home. At first, during the lockdown, I was able to keep my wig curled and styled. As time went on, I had to be a little creative. I began pulling it back into a ponytail, and eventually wore pretty scarves for accessories and to keep my wig securely on. In the end, I even wore a headband around my wig to keep it on. The fear of not wanting to see what my head looked like underneath my wig was overwhelming to me. I was so happy when the order was lifted, I got a chance to go back into the salon to let Ms. Stephanie care for my hair again.

Pamela W

 I have been losing my hair for the majority of my adult life. I am considered middle-aged, but I still have a zest for life and a desire to look good. I have been a client of Trinity Lace Wigs, and its owner Ms. Anderson, for close to 13 years now. The COVID-19 shelter-in-place mandate did not apply to me. My job is considered essential, I work in the healthcare industry and was on the front lines practically every day during the height of the pandemic. I love my job and I love serving the community.

I knew firsthand how important it was to abide by the closure of what was considered "non-essential" businesses, which included Ms. Anderson's wig shop. What I learned about myself during that time of her closure was the level of denial I was in. Since she has been taking care of my hair, I don't have to do barely anything to my hair. All of a sudden, I was responsible for taking care of it all by myself. It was scary for me.

Ms. Anderson was there with me on the phone, rooting me on and giving me the encouragement, I needed. When I took my wig off, I don't think she heard the sadness I was experiencing. I always try to be the glass is "half full" person. It had been years since I have seen my hair loss, and having to see the totality of it, and how much it had spread was sobering. I locked myself in the bathroom, all by myself, breaking my heart. I am so used to having hair. The wigs that Ms. Anderson provides to me and styles for me, I consider it my own hair. After so many years of wearing it, it looks so real that I consider it as my own. The true fact was having to come to grips with it. I wasn't prepared, but I did it.

I can't remember, but it was like 3 months before her place reopened, and during that time it became easier and easier for me to manage. I even had her order me a new wig. This time, she made me a personal video and sent it to me on how to cut the lace without damaging it. I did my best with it. Granted, I can't make my wig do what she makes it do, but I am glad I was able to care for myself when she wasn't able to.

I know Ms. Anderson was brokenhearted that she couldn't be there for me, and the rest of her clients, during her brief closure. She wasn't there physically, but she was there in other ways; and I am so glad because she really cares for her clients. This experience has proven to me that I can take care of myself if I need to, but I could not wait until the shelter-in-place orders were removed.

Taking Nothing for Granted

The truth of the matter is, I did not know how some of my clients were going to fare through the 13-week mandated closure of my facility during the peak of COVID-19. A vast majority of them do not want to think about their hair loss, do not want to look at their hair loss, and do not identify with their hair loss. They practice other coping mechanisms that allow them to get through having hair loss.

I engage with them and always try to provide that listening ear, coach, and encourage them. What I do above all else is reinforce self-confidence, self-worth, and the beauty within each of them regardless of how "follicly" challenged they are. Many of them came to me from major "big" boy industry corporations; some came from mom-and-pop hair replacement centers. These facilities made them feel like they were just a number, or had them so convinced that "no one else" knew how to do hair replacement; they were stuck with whatever treatment, products and/or services they provided.

Clients Have Choices

I take nothing for granted. When my ministry of hair replacement found me, I immediately learned the weight of responsibility of what I would be taking on. Unlike my many years as a stylist, there are tear-jerking realities that many do not consider when working with clients facing the lifelong journey of hair loss.

Secrets and Spouses

Sophie was a client to whom I had been providing services for six (6) years at that time. One day during an appointment, she reminded me that her 26th wedding anniversary was in a few weeks. She recounted some special memories with her husband and even shared with me how they met. Imagine, fast-forward, close to 26 years of marriage is almost upon them. She talked about how he made her tingle every time he looked at her, how after all these years, they still complete each other's sentences, how they share everything with one another...well, not everything.

She looked sad, she said she believes he knows there's "something" going on with her hair, but she has never talked about losing her hair with him. He has never seen her without her hair system on. After all of these years with my client and husband having shared so much together, it hit me. This is her life partner, her soul mate, the man she loves, trusts, and shares intimate moments with. She has a personal issue that she has not revealed to him, but has entrusted me to provide care and service to and for her. It is real. It is emotional. It is something that cannot, and must not be taken for granted, or advantage of. The responsibility of caring for this special demographic of clients has been, and still is, one of the most rewarding parts of my career in beauty.

* * *

Male Fascination with Hair

Do men really just find long hair attractive on women for no apparent reason? Of course, there are those who do not because you cannot assign a belief system to any one group and say "everybody". However, there are a great many men who do.

Sure, we get it. The majority of men prefer women with long hair. Primitive, or so the theory goes. If a caveman saw a woman he fancied, he could simply take her by the hair and carry her off. I know that sounds funny, but it's true.

A man who tried such caveman techniques on his wife, girlfriend, significant other, or any woman today would likely face jail time, if not worse. However, the mentality underlying such activities hasn't changed much over the centuries. Men prefer women with longer hair because it emphasizes their femininity and makes them seem more distinct from men.

The Hidden Truth

The nurse called for Mrs. Smith, who waved goodbye to her husband of 22 years as he waited for her return in the reception area. As she sat in the exam room of the dermatology clinic, she began to remember just how she got there.

She remembered a small, irregularly shaped growth on her scalp that appeared out of nowhere seven years ago. Concerned it may be a cancerous growth, she got it tested. A biopsy revealed it was a nevus, a simple mole. However, as the years went by, she noticed some obvious hair thinning in that area, and the mole began to spread. She decided to have it removed. The size of the area left her with no choice but to have a scalp reduction.

The doctor assured Gladys that the remaining hairs surrounding that area were healthy and her follicles would not be compromised. In the years since her procedure, her hair loss has become substantial. She was hoping to find out why she was losing her hair.

Thankfully, her doctor specializes in skin and scalp maladies and works with women with hair loss. She was diagnosed with a scarring type of alopecia and discovered that the Polycystic Ovarian Syndrome (PCOS) that went undiagnosed for 5 years may have led to some of her thinning hair. She did not realize that it was possible to have more than one type of hair loss issue.

After her appointment, she knew that she must address her hair loss with Mr. Smith. The drive home was pleasant. Her husband was curious but dared not pry. He'd been with her long enough to know that when she was ready to share her thoughts, she would.

Gladys decided to talk to her husband over dinner and address the elephant in the room. She made his favorite meal, and they shared a little casual conversation about their day.

Mrs. Smith has always taken pride in her appearance. She believed in self-care, keeping standing appointments for her facials, manicures, massages, and weekly appointments to make sure her wig was perfectly styled. There was a point in her life when wearing a wig was a want, but now it had turned into a need.

During dessert, she began one of the most personal and vulnerable conversations with her husband, detailing her hair loss. As beautiful as she believed herself to be to him, she already knew what his reaction to her would be. He was understanding and supportive.

Mr. Smith knew something was going on with his wife, as she had begun to change her beauty regimen around him regarding her hair. She was either always wearing a wig, a scarf, or some type of head covering around him.

Mrs. Smith dropped the question, "Do you want to see my hair loss?" to her husband. He replied, "No, I do not." She shared everything with her husband, yet she needed to know why he did not want to see her hair loss. She recounted Mr. Smith's explanation that, ever since he'd known her, she had hair. He ran his fingers through her hair on many occasions. He did not want to see her hair loss or the scar. He does not want to see if it gets worse. He thought it might turn him off. He will support her with her medical appointments, and he will go wig shopping with her; he will help her choose her wigs and even pay for them. He did not doubt that she would continue to take care of her appearance and that she would always be attractive to him. "I do not want to see anything that would mess up that image of you for me," he shared.

Then she did it; she let out an audible exhale. The hidden truth is that it had taken years for Gladys to come out of denial about this very personal situation. When it was no longer avoidable and there was an actual diagnosis along with her very visible situation, she felt obligated to share it with her husband. She loves the way he looks at her and how he shows her affection, and he has no problem with PDA even after all of these years. Mrs. Smith never wants her husband to look at her any differently. Although her offer never included her public reveal, her love and adoration for her husband inclined her to share with him. She hated having to keep the secret. She is uncomfortable with her situation, but as time goes on, even this may change. However, for right now, she has accepted her loss.

Mrs. Smith's hair loss has gotten a lot worse. Mr. Smith still shows so much adoration toward his wife. Whenever Mrs. Smith closes the bathroom door in their home, Mr. Smith has never walked in on her. He gives her space to work on various at-home scalp treatments; he still takes her to her hair appointments with her trichologist to treat her scalp and care for her natural hair underneath her wigs. They do have a loving relationship, but after all these years of going through her gradual hair loss, he still has not seen her balding scalp.

Some may say she is hiding underneath her wig. She doesn't believe that to be the case. Sharing with the person who means the most to her was her utmost concern. What the world at large thinks about her, if anything at all, is of no consequence. There is no obligation to prove anything to anyone.

I intentionally took a little additional time when capturing the experience of my client, Ms. Gladys. I wish you could envision her. She is a mature, professional woman who works in corporate America and enjoys paying attention to the details of caring for her home and family. She is by no means a shrinking violet. I watched her recall those difficult moments as she shared her experience with me. Her eyes spoke louder than her eloquence in speech and voice.

Regardless of your experience with hair loss or alopecia, whether it affects you, someone you care about, or just a casual acquaintance, you must know that it is personal and emotional.

* * *

Have I not commanded you? Be strong and courageous. Do not be frightened, and do not be dismayed, for the Lord your God is with you wherever you go. *Joshua 1:9 (ESV)*

CHAPTER 9

PSYCHOLOGY AND HAIR LOSS

Is There Bald Bias?

Are there people with biases against hair loss and bald heads? Is there a subconscious message that people with hair thinning, loss, or balding heads are inferior, less desirable, and less beautiful? Hair standards are normalized in a variety of ways within a greater culture of beauty. The beauty business influences our visual intake on a daily basis, thanks to editorials, advertising, fashion, Hollywood, and social media. Because our impressions are mostly based on implicit visual processes, continuous exposure to smooth, silky, full, and voluminous hair associated with beauty, popularity, and riches generates the connection that a bountiful head of hair is the beauty default.

Given what I know about other types of bias, I'm curious how widespread bald bias affects views of attractiveness, self-esteem, sense of professionalism; and by extension, career possibilities for persons whose follicular challenges differ from the norm. Unfortunately, I won't be able to go into detail in this writing about unfavorable stereotypes or attitudes about those who have hair loss, whether unconsciously or consciously.

In the meantime, consider the following questions to assess your own biases—knowing these will help you understand your

ALOPECIA, IT'S A THING! BREAKING THROUGH THE B.S. (BELIEF SYSTEMS)

worldview. As a coach, I must be objective and non-judgmental; therefore, it was critical for me to be honest with myself. I'm sharing this exercise with you because many individuals don't realize it until they are confronted with difficult questions. There are common biases in the following categories—do you have strong feelings, preferences, or dislikes for any of the following categories? (Note your answers below):

Age:

Religion:

Sexuality:

Gender:

Beauty/Hair:

Skin-tone:

Weight:

Ethnicity:

Race:

Disabilities:

Other:

If you are not sure if you have any biases in these categories, find out by taking the Implicit Association Test here: https:// implicit.harvard.edu/impli cit/takeatest.ht

Peladophobia (Fear of Bald People)

Have you ever felt that people are staring at or avoiding you? It's possible that you are not imagining it. Although not very common, it is a condition called Peladophobia. This condition is very real. There is an actual phobia or fear of bald people.

Peladophobia is the name for the irrational fear of bald people. Even thinking about bald people, let alone seeing one, can cause extreme anxiety in someone with this condition. In fact, their anxiety can be so intense that it might even give them a full-blown panic attack. For those who have peladophobia, that will not always be the case, but it is still very likely that such an onslaught of fear will occur.

In addition to other symptoms, a person experiencing a full-blown panic attack due to peladophobia should prepare for a rise in blood pressure, heart rate, breathing rate, blood pressure, muscle tension, trembling, and profuse sweating. Although not everyone who has peladophobia may suffer panic attacks, it is nevertheless possible, particularly if their symptoms are very extreme.

The condition is not described as having anxiety or fear about becoming bald, like most people. This phobia is associated with those who have bald heads. Like many phobias, those with it are overly scared of the fear's trigger. In this case, someone with extreme hair loss, even when a person is aware of the fear's irrationality, they are powerless over it.

Which is More Dangerous?

If you meet someone who is trying to give you "toxic praise" or someone who is trying to "avoid you at all costs" out of fear, you might wonder which is the more dangerous of the two.

For me personally, what matters most is intent. Possibly my rationale comes from my previous training as a paralegal or from watching too many court shows on television. I believe, for general intent, in law. It only needs to be proven that the perpetrator, "toxic praise" or "peladophobia", intended to do the act in question. Considering that proving specific intent would require that the perpetrator, "toxic praise" or "peladophobia", intended to bring about a specific consequence through their actions or that they performed the action with a wrongful purpose. My take on it is that the "toxic praise" person's definition means they intend to use praise for manipulative purposes to elicit hurtful feelings in the person with hair loss. Whereas, the person with "peladophobia" retreats from interacting with the person with hair loss. They may elicit hurtful feelings, but there is no intent because their actions are motivated by uncontrollable fear rather than malice.

No matter what anyone's intention was, the person with hair loss or baldness is affected if they feel bad about themselves because of it. This could lead to lack of confidence, low self-esteem, embarrassment, anxiety, etc.

Gloriously Bald

Every year on September 13, people celebrate "National Bald is Beautiful Day." Although it is a U.S. holiday, we believe it should be observed globally! Many people experience fear and humiliation as a result of being bald. It's nothing to be ashamed of though! Both having hair and being bald are extremely common in nature. "National Bald is Beautiful Day" serves as a gentle reminder that everyone, bald or not, is beautiful in their own unique way. September 13, is the day to compliment your bald buddies on their beauty. The goal of the festivities is to spread joy.

Although for some, coping with thinning hair, moderate hair loss, and/or baldness is extremely difficult, there are others who embrace their baldness and are confident in the beauty they possess inside as well as outside. Here are the words of one such beauty, who shares her journey on Facebook posts using #BaldWhisperer.

My story:

 In June 2020 my hair started falling out in patches. At that stage, we credited stress and medication, for unrelated issues, as the factors and I cut my hair shorter. In March 2021, the patches started again. I was diagnosed with Alopecia Areata. I had no other choice than to shave my hair off, completely. I have since lost hair on my right arm and eyebrows also. If I tell you my hair loss experience was easy, I would definitely be lying. I was standing in my bathroom, shaver ready in my hand, staring at myself in the big mirror. I was angry, frustrated, crying, and angry again. I bent over the bath and shaved my hair off. When I came up, with a tear-streaked face and raccoon eyes, I saw my reflection and bald head in the mirror and I remember thinking, "Oh wow, I have a beautiful head!" From there on, I had peace with my shaved head.

Alopecia Areata occurs when the immune system attacks hair follicles, an auto-immune disease, resulting in sudden hair loss that starts with one or more circular bald patches. So, in short, the only thing tough enough to kick my butt is me! I may have lost my hair but not my sense of humor.

There is no cure for Alopecia and it's not considered a serious medical condition, but it can cause a lot of anxiety and sadness. It may not be life-threatening, but it is life-altering.

By telling my story, I hope to educate people about Alopecia and try to break the "perfect look" stereotype that we get slammed with daily. I want to show people that we are all perfect just the way we are because beauty comes from within. I want to encourage others, who might feel different, that although I have a big, shiny, bald head, who I am is much more important than what I look like. I refuse to let this disease take my self-esteem. When you have Alopecia and you feel like you are alone, let go of that feeling and get in contact with me. Behind every bald head is a powerful story, one worth changing someone else's life.

What I can tell you about being bald?

1. It's very neat, not a hair out of place!

2. I can style my hair with a damp washcloth!

3. The more hair I lose, the more head I get.

4. I do take longer to wash my face now...

Telling me "It's just hair", is not helping in the slightest. I wish it was just hair, but it's not. According to society, it's the picture of how a woman should look like. For me, it was the difference between feeling attractive or not, the difference between feeling OK or avoiding leaving the house, and the difference between having my confidence shattered or someone not being comfortable seeing my bald head. It affects you on a daily basis.

When my hair started falling out, it was PAINFUL! My scalp was on fire, tender, and sore. Even now, as soon as I experience a "flare up", I can actually tell by the burning sensation exactly where the next bald spot will appear. It feels like I can boil a packet of frozen peas, during load shedding til perfection, in a matter of minutes. Wigs, hats, and scarves were definitely never an option for me because of the tenderness. For different people, it happens differently. There is no cure but there are various treatments available. But for me, I decided to be gloriously bald, cracked, worn, and dented because I've never heard of a clean, shiny sword that ever won a war, and me...I'm ready for battle!

Caren Venter, South Africa

Alopecia Warriors

There are countless Alopecia Warriors who have been drafted into this battle with hair loss; they did not voluntarily enlist. However, many of them see and feel the "battle scars" and are war-weary. Like most things in life, the effects are different for everyone.

Many women feel as if they have been dropped into a war zone with very little support or ammunition to combat the enemy. They need help and resources.

 Angel R. successfully beat breast cancer. In February 2019, she felt a lump in her breast. So, she did the smart thing and had a routine check. Angel went to see her gynecologist, a wonderful doctor in her hometown.

Due to her age, he initially suspected fibroids when examining her. He felt that it wasn't anything serious, but thank God he did not rely on that. Her gynecologist wanted to be sure, so he scheduled a mammogram for her, followed by an ultrasound, which led to a biopsy. The result was breast cancer.

Her prognosis was good. She did get a second opinion, which reinforced the initial diagnosis as well as the proposed therapy regimen following her oncologist's advice and treatment. She was cancer-free! During her 5 months of treatment, she experienced very little hair shedding or hair loss. It wasn't easy, but she did it!

Fast-forward to summer 2022. Angel sent me a Facebook message. It is a picture of Angel's scalp; she's afraid, her hair is falling out, and she has two smooth circular patches of her scalp exposed; each the size of a quarter, one in the top crown and the other near the nape of her neck. As she had recently moved back to her hometown, I recommended a colleague near her. I was familiar with the signs and symptoms of Alopecia Areata (AA); however, I wanted to give her the opportunity to sit down with a trichologist who would be able to perform a more thorough consultation and assessment.

Indeed, she was diagnosed with AA. Within two months, the number and size of the spots increased. She was devastated. She beat breast cancer, and although her hair follicles were resilient through cancer treatment, they were no match for this new autoimmune disease, alopecia areata.

I recommended that she work with the trichologist and seek counseling to reinforce her emotional state. A few days later, I learned she had decided to shave her entire head. Initially, she felt so liberated. Her confidence, which she shared, fluctuated. She does not identify with her self-worth being associated with her hair. We all know that it is not, right?

Her struggles came from the stares, the whispers, the pointing, and the negative comments from others. As a single woman, she has experienced men flat-out avoiding her and just being rude. The difference is obvious in treatment before and after hair loss. She has begun to question her decision and feels vulnerable.

Drop the Zeros

It's unavoidable not to mention the double standard between men and women. A man losing his hair and going completely bald is more socially acceptable than a woman experiencing the same loss or hair challenges. Now, whether or not that man losing his hair is ready to accept his Level 7 degrees of loss on the Norwood Hair Loss Chart is another matter and possibly another book all together.

However, not much would be said in society about him. Even some may think he looks more handsome, distinguished, or debonair without his hair. You'd be hard-pressed to hear many, if any, positive descriptors about the fairer sex losing her hair.

My personal opinion is that we all have a certain set of criteria that we find attractive in others. Many can be superficial, lack depth, and are shallow; but to each their own, unless it is harmful to others. Growing up, I was attracted to nicely cut or closely faded shaven styles in men. Never had I considered dating, much less marrying, anyone without hair. When I met my husband, he was already shaving his head completely bald. He was and is so handsome that, over time, I fell in love and never gave it a second thought. If the roles were reversed, I cannot honestly say that would be the issue for many men meeting a woman with substantial hair loss.

Contrary to that, I have found that those already in a committed relationship tend to be less judgmental or superficial toward their partner if they lose their hair during the relationship. Similarly, losing your hair is like losing other appendages of the body. If you were to suffer a major illness or lose an eye, arm, leg, etc., would your significant other feel any differently about you or love you any less?

A similar question is asked later through surveys in Chapter 11. The answer with regard to those respondents varies in accordance with their marital or relationship status. Searching online, I came across a forum discussion of the question, "Do men find bald women unattractive?" (quora.com/Do-men-find-bald-women-unattractive). The discussion had varying opinions:

1. Respondent – Prometheus (male) "I want to give a very clear answer here. Of course, I love seeing waist length hair on a woman. BUT If, God forbid, something happened to an intimate partner that caused her to lose her hair? It would never make me not love someone anymore. That would be the height of "_____" to abandon a lover for something she had no control over."

2. Respondent – Mike R (male) "Absolutely! VERY UNATTRACTIVE! Now on the other hand if the women has cancer or another medical issue, I understand and feel compassionate for them."

3. Respondent – Ted Morgan (male) "I find bald girls extraordinarily appealing..."

4. Respondent – Amy Oakes (female) "I had to shave for cancer. The majority of people I knew told me it looked good, but I'm sure it looked awful. I know I have the perfect headshape for it, but massive hot water scars on my scalp are not pretty. I noticed the sexual attention I received whilst bald dropped. And still with short hair, its very low. You rarely get harassed or catcalled. Its quite nice actually. Very peaceful. A few men I know admitted having massive fetishes for bald, a la Sigourney Weaver. It was only a few guys though. A rare fetish. And if I create two identical Tinder accounts, one bald, one with a wig; u can guess which one gets the matches. Long hair is just a traditional symbol of femininity."

As you can see, very individual and varying opinions emerged from different respondents to the same question. Everyone is entitled to their feelings and opinions, and this is true. No one, however, should be made to feel less than human or of less value by someone else. If someone is making you feel this way, ditch the zero and find a hero.

Opposing Struggles

So, is it just me, or does there seem to be a little tension between the "no hair, don't care"—I will not cover my head and the "no hair, I don't dare"—I will always wear a wig, I must cover my head, groups? With the hair loss community rapidly expanding, there appears to be an uproar of opinions on how people should present themselves in the world. Whether they are exposing or not exposing their scalps, I have been in conversations with those on both sides.

Those women who have embraced their hair loss and their baldness display them like a beautiful and majestic badge of honor. I remember a quote from Representative Ayanna Pressley, "I don't need hair to have a crown", a very noteworthy and self-empowering mantra. She has undoubtedly been helpful in being one of the faces of alopecia and initiating the conversation on hair loss.

In addition to those women, there is a large group of people for whom I provide care. Due to their hair loss, they will wear the most beautiful hair via wigs, prostheses, hair units, and various head coverings. They are mortified at the notion of exposing their heads and scalps to the general public. They have the very best and most beautifully coiffed wigs and hair pieces to wear and express themselves with.

Recently, I had a conversation with someone who called me about their diagnosed autoimmune condition, Alopecia Totalis (AT). She made the decision to not wear wigs almost immediately after losing all of her hair. She is taking control of her hair loss in her own way. I was somewhat taken aback by her statement against other women with hair loss who cover up their deficiencies using wigs, hair pieces, hats, etc. She mentioned the sacrifices she and others like her are making by being the true face of Alopecia.

Yet, on the other end of the spectrum, countless women with Alopecia have questioned why women would choose not to cover their scalps. Personally, they could not fathom not wearing hair. For them, that's how they control their loss.

Either way, what a person chooses to do is a personal choice. There is no right, and there is no wrong. It just is. What may work for one person may not work for another, or the masses. Everyone has different comfort levels, and I support people in doing what feels right for them.

These stances of opposition are dealing with the same struggle: Hair Loss! It saddens me. It reminds me of the commentary I used to read regarding natural vs. relaxed hair. As women, our hair is a sensitive and frequently over-discussed topic of conversation and debate. It's hurtful and divisive.

As a professional who has dedicated my profession to assisting women with hair loss, it grieves me. I don't take sides. I provide beautiful hair alternatives to those who want them. These gorgeous ladies, whether they want a short, conservative bob or 30 inches down their back, can have whatever they want. I got her. At the same time, I make sure to attend to the health of the scalps of those beauties who want to rock their bald heads by providing scalp therapy treatments. That's what I do.

If you hear nothing else, I say please hear this. Love each other, and don't judge each other. As women, we must love and accept people where they are.

Self Esteem

Proverbs 23:7 For as a man thinketh in his heart, so is he

There are questions we might ask ourselves when we think about self-esteem. What is the definition of self-esteem? How is it developed? What constitutes good or bad self-esteem? Can bad self-esteem be changed into a healthier one? The definition of self-esteem is basically how a person sees him or herself. Your self-esteem is made up of thoughts and feelings that have been shaped since childhood. Your level of self-esteem is based on unique experiences, both good and bad, and personal relationships that have impacted your life. Self-esteem is shaped by relationships formed in childhood with adults and friends, sports, clubs, hobbies, and teams. It has an impact on your relationships with your spouse, parents, grandparents, brothers and sisters, classmates, employers, and coworkers, to name a few. Know that positive experiences help to raise your level of self-esteem. When you value the type of person you are, you have a good concept of high self-esteem. You are proud to be you; you value your skills and talents, and respect your intelligence. You also act on your beliefs and feelings and accept the person you are.

Feeling good about yourself is another way to say you have high self-esteem. It is not egotism or snobbishness. There is not one single event or person that can determine your level of self-esteem. It evolves over time and is constantly influenced by experience. High self-esteem enables you to accept challenges, enrich your life, maintain self-confidence, and remain flexible. You are not afraid to develop your abilities or to trust; you are more willing to take risks and try new things. Trying new things is how you grow; if you do not try, you will not grow. You can become stuck in a pattern of negative thoughts; you may presume the worst about things.

Self-esteem affects the way we live. Remember, we all want to be accepted; we want to be "OK." You can be a conduit to help others around you feel better about themselves. Self-esteem involves how we think, act, and feel, not only about ourselves but also others. Some examples of high self-esteem are: "I am pretty," "I am smart," "I learn from my mistakes," and "I am fun to be around." Self-esteem can also determine how successful you are at achieving goals. High self-esteem can make you feel effective, productive, capable, and loveable. With high self-esteem, you are a joy to be around. By being happier with yourself, you will be eager to meet new friends and develop closer relationships.

When you maintain self-confidence, remember that believing you can do something is half the battle. You can stand against the odds. You learn to give yourself wholeheartedly to whatever you are doing, and it does not matter if you win or lose. High self-esteem does not guarantee success, but it does guarantee feeling good about yourself and others.

We all know that change is not easy and can be frightening and unfamiliar at times. You learn to face your fears. Having a positive self-image makes it easier to accept new ideas and ways of doing things. With high self-esteem, you have a "can do" attitude, and you take pride in yourself. Also, know that a positive attitude rubs off on others around you. Offering encouragement, being patient with others and yourself, and not pointing out others' faults and weaknesses--everyone has them, it exhibits a positive attitude. You make it a point to be your own best friend, and you identify and accept your strengths and weaknesses.

Everyone wants to be accepted, and low self-esteem says that you are not "OK". Something is wrong with you, and you gravitate towards the negative. Negative self-esteem robs you of your self-worth; it is the opposite of high self-esteem. It distorts your view of yourself and others. With low self-esteem, you think others are better than you. The more you dwell on the negative, the lower your self-esteem gets. Low self-esteem can make you feel ineffective, worthless, incompetent, and unloved. When you lack self-confidence, you tend to feel that you are doomed to fail. Therefore, fear sets in, and you become stuck in a downward spiral of negative thought patterns. Poor performance is another sign of low self-esteem; you tend to make little or no effort toward realizing projects or goals. With low self-esteem, you can be unhappy with your personal life. Some people may find it hard to develop close relationships. Some people isolate themselves, which can cause loneliness. For healing, you must learn to interrupt these negative thought patterns. Instead of seeing yourself as "ugly, stupid, afraid to fail, boring," etc., you change your self-talk. "I am beautiful." There is only one other person like me in the world. Tell yourself repeatedly that "I am smart", "I am not afraid to fail". Explore the gifts and abilities that God has given you. In the Bible, in Philippians 4:8, it says, "Finally, brethren, whatsoever things are true, whatsoever things are honest, whatsoever things are just, whatsoever things are pure, whatsoever things are lovely, whatsoever things are of a good report; if there be any virtue, and if there be any praise, think on these things."

This change does not happen overnight, but change takes time. You must learn to love and respect yourself for who you are. You must learn to trust yourself and pay attention to your thoughts and feelings. You will gradually act on what you think is right. You will learn to do what makes you happy, and you will tend to view yourself differently. You believe that God created you with a purpose and loves you just the way you are. Therefore, I encourage you to take a hard look at yourself and then change the things about you that you do not like. You have a lifetime to do this, but the results will be well worth the effort. Consulting a counselor may help you on this journey.

Carolyn Stovall, B.A. in Psychology and Sociology and a minor in Women's Studies from Bellevue College (Bellevue, Nebraska). She also has a Master's in Community Counseling from St. Mary's University (San Antonio, Texas).

* * *

God is within her, she will not fall; God will help her at break of day. *Psalms 46:5 (NIV)*

CHAPTER 10

ONE DAY AT A TIME

Doesn't Happen Overnight

D espite the fact that circumstances in life can change quickly, people however tend to do so more slowly. Even God took six (6) days to create the Earth and everything in it. When you consider the progression from general to more complex as God created the Earth's ecosystem, the six days make logical sense. For it to be documented in the book of Genesis and for us to see the rationale, strength, insight, and discipline of God in creation, it's possible that God was demonstrating wisdom by taking the time to arrange everything in order over extended periods of time.

So, do not feel like you have to change the way you are feeling and the insecurities about your hair loss instantaneously. Change does not happen overnight; it takes time. If you can take one day at a time to practice building your self-esteem and self-confidence, you can make a difference in your life. In Proverbs 18:21 (NIV), it states, "The tongue has the power of life and death, and those who love it will eat its fruit." Practice speaking love, life, and goodness over yourself with positive affirmations, quotes, songs, etc.

Positive Affirmations

Your body changes physiologically in reaction to the ideas that go through your mind each moment of every day. Your brain sends signals and releases neurotransmitters simply by thinking about something. Almost all of your body's processes, including your emotions and moods, are controlled by these chemicals. Affirmations, also known as self-affirmations, are ideas you consciously think in order to strengthen, inspire, and relax your mind and body. They can be uplifting assertions that are used to contradict pessimistic, depressive, or anxiety-inducing ideas and attitudes. They might simply be sentiments of general encouragement and support. You can use affirmations to change your moods, thought patterns, and behavioral routines.

Create Your Own Affirmations

Your affirmations will be personalized to you and the goals, changes, or issues you desire to address. You can modify the examples below to reflect your specific needs. Affirmations work best when you repeat them to yourself frequently and as needed. It's helpful to repeat them throughout the day, for instance, when you have unfavorable thoughts, feelings, or come into difficult emotional circumstances. You should breathe slowly and deeply while using affirmations. Concentrate on the affirmation and the feelings that go along with it as you are aware of your breath coming in and going out of you.

It is For Everyone

Positive affirmations for self-esteem sounds like they should only be used when a person lacks self-confidence; but in truth, you can use them whenever you want to feel better about yourself or need a confidence boost. Try a few:

- I am enough just as I am

- I am beautiful

- I am a woman designed divinely by God to be feminine, and I am

- I am unique

- I am beautiful and perfect just the way I am

- I am worthy of love

- There is no such thing as an ugly woman

- Life is beautiful

- I am perfect just as I am, today

- The things in my life are just incredible opportunities for growth and challenge when I encounter them

- I deserve happiness and success

- I am not my hair, or lack thereof

- Good morning beautiful

- I cherish all that is beautiful concerning me, including my flaws just as much as my strengths

- I am beautiful, no matter what

- No one has the power to define me but me

- I love how confident I feel when my mind is focused, clear and relaxed

- My inner beauty is what allows me to stand out in a crowd

- I'm grateful for my insecurities because they make me strive harder

Try these — https://positiveaffirmationscenter.com/positive-affirmations-for-women/

Here is also a short list of songs that I'd like to recommend that may encourage and empower you. If nothing else, the beat to a few of them is excellent to workout to!

1. "Better Than Good" by *Todd Galberth*

2. "Changing Your Story" by *Jekalyn Carr*

3. "Good Morning Gorgeous" by *Mary J. Blige*

4. "God In Me" by *Mary Mary*

5. "You Are So Beautiful" by *Joe Cocker* (version – CK Gospel Choir)

6. "I Am Not My Hair" by *India Arie*

7. Stronger (What Doesn't Kill You)" by *Kelly Clarkson*

8. "Unpretty" by *TLC*

9. "Whip My Hair Back and Forth" by *Willow Smith*

10. "It Keeps Happening" by *Kierra Sheard*

These are just a few from my playlist, and yes, they're eclectic. I believe personally, music is food for the soul; listen to what ministers to you and inspires you. I am sure you have a few favorite songs you love that motivate and make you feel special and invincible. Those are the songs that you need when you begin to feel "less than" and begin to question your self-worth. You are more than a conqueror. Just make an effort each day; take it one day at a time!

Please do me a favor—let me know if you have a favorite affirmation, quote, or song. Like the AlopeciaItsAThing page on FB; and comment or email me at AlopeciaItsAThing@gmail. I'd love to hear from you.

Over the years, I have helped many clients with hair loss. As you know, alopecia, or hair loss, is one of those topics that, depending on who you are, elicits a variety of reactions. If you do not experience hair loss, it is probable that you do not worry about it. However, if you are one of the millions of individuals who do, it may be on your mind constantly. Alopecia can affect just your scalp or the entire body, and it can be either transient or permanent. Hereditary reasons, hormonal changes, illnesses, or a normal part of aging could all contribute to it. Hair loss, and the numerous changes it causes, can happen to anyone.

Developing Your Alopecia Support Squad (A$$)

In your journey with alopecia, from time to time, you may feel the need to talk with someone. Talk about your feelings, emotions, challenges, or even someone to celebrate your victories and milestones with. To prepare for those times, I want to share some ideas on how to get some women allies to support you. Here are a few suggestions for how to put together a group of go-to girls.

Any individuals who come together with the goal of supporting one another while coping with alopecia is considered an "Alopecia Support Squad". The size of a support group may vary—it could be tiny, a casual meeting at someone's kitchen table; or big, a group at an Alopecia Awareness assembly, or in the meeting room of a religious organization. Participants may come from a particular segment of the alopecia community, women, children, or men with alopecia. Some candidates may be caregivers of those living with alopecia, members of a faith community, or anyone who wishes to attend and discuss alopecia and its emotional implications.

1. Determine the frequency of meetings and where: Weekly, Monthly, or Quarterly at different homes

2. Decide the mission of your support group. This will serve as your anchor and whom you invite to the group. It also answers why it exists.

3. Give thought to the group invitees. Make sure everyone can get along comfortably and safely. Keep the group intimate.

4. Determine what you want to accomplish: support, encouragement, volunteer, etc.

5. Keep everyone motivated.

National Support Groups/Resources

1. National Alopecia Areata Foundation

2. Coalition of Skin Diseases

3. American Academy of Dermatology Association

4. Alopecia World

Social Media – Facebook has multiple groups, just search and join!

In this book, I pray that regardless of who you are and what your experience is with alopecia, you have found some valuable information contained within the covers of this book. Remember, I care about you.

Please review my book to help me connect with more people struggling with alopecia. I desperately want them to know that they are not alone, that they are not the only ones, and that I am here to encourage them. I desire in providing tools and resources to assist them along their journey with hair loss.

Be sure to visit **www.AlopeciaItsAThing.com** and sign up to get updates on my projects about hair loss.

* * *

For we are God's masterpiece. He has created us anew in Christ Jesus, so we can do the good things he planned for us long ago. *Ephesians 2:10 (NLV)*

CHAPTER 11

SOCIAL EXPERIMENT AND SURVEYS

Social Experiment – Bald Head Filter

T here are those who constantly have hair loss on their minds because they live with it every day. There are others who may not have ever considered what it would look or feel like to have alopecia. Hear from a small sampling of women without hair loss who see themselves through a "bald" app and PhotoShopped photos. The following pages contain the unedited and actual responses of this survey from a selection of them:

Respondent #1

Is it OK to use your name, or any identifying information, in print? Yes, it is OK.

First name (or initial): Veronica.

Last name (or initial): D.

How old are you? 25-34

What was your first thought upon seeing yourself with a bald head? I'm still beautiful.

Please rate the following statement: "A woman's hair is her crown and glory": 1 = Strongly Agree, 2 = Generally Agree,

3 = Somewhat Disagree, 4 = Strongly Disagree, 5 = I am not sure/Not Applicable, 3 = Somewhat Disagree.

Do you think if you had alopecia, hair loss, would it change the way you see yourself and live your life? I think it would definitely affect my self-esteem, but not the way I live my life.

If you are in a relationship, would your significant other understand and accept you with hair loss? Would there be a change in the way your partner would see or treat you? Yes, he would. I lived with postpartum hair loss and shaved my head as an outcome of the hair loss.

Prior to seeing this image of yourself, have you ever thought about what if you lost your hair? Yes.

Have you ever had an opinion, positive or negative, about seeing a woman with hair loss? Yes.

If so, to the above question, please explain: I always wondered what happened to cause the baldness, was it choices, was it medical, etc.

Would you be willing to share your photo or video screenshot of your bald head filter? Yes

If you had to pick between a beautiful head of healthy hair or your dream career, which would be more important to you? Why? My dream career. Hair can be bought, dreams can't.

Would you like to add or share any additional information and thoughts to this survey? No.

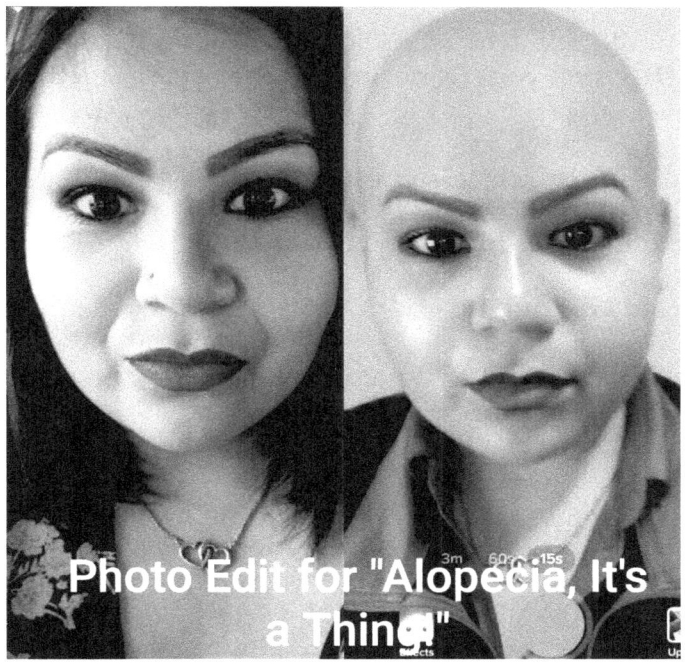

Veronica "Bald App" Photo to Replicate Bald Head

Respondent #2

Is it OK to use your name, or any identifying information, in print? Yes, it is OK.

First name (or initial): Nikke.

Last name (or initial): B.

How old are you? 25-34.

What was your first thought upon seeing yourself with a bald head? I'm still beautiful.

Please rate the following statement: "A woman's hair is her crown and glory": 1 = Strongly Agree, 2 = Generally Agree, 3 = Somewhat Disagree, 4 = Strongly Disagree, 5 = I am not sure/Not Applicable 2 = Generally Agree.

Do you think if you had alopecia, hair loss, would it change the way you see yourself and live your life? Yes, I believe that it would.

If you're in a relationship, would your significant other understand and accept you with hair loss? Would there be a change in the way your partner would see or treat you? He would 100% understand and treat me no different.

Prior to seeing this image of yourself, have you ever thought about what if you lost your hair? Yes.

Have you ever had an opinion, positive or negative, about seeing a woman with hair loss? Yes.

If so, to the above question, please explain: I always say I think of how strong they are and their confidence, the testimony and story behind their hair loss.

Would you be willing to share your photo or video screenshot of your bald head filter? Yes.

If you had to pick between a beautiful head of healthy hair or your dream career, which would be more important to you? Why? Dream career is more important to me because my hair is a feature of my physical appearance; but it doesn't prevent me from accomplishing any of my dreams.

Would you like to add or share any additional information and thoughts to this survey? No

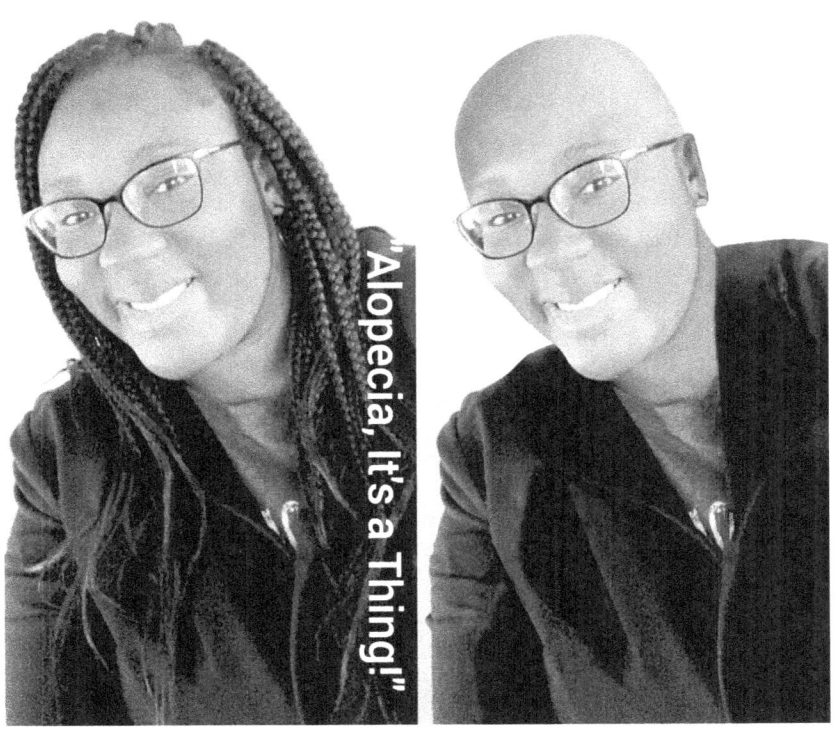

Nikke "PhotoShopped" Photo to Replicate Bald Head

Respondent #3

Is it OK to use your name, or any identifying information, in print? Yes, it is OK.

First name (or initial): Yolanda.

Last name (or initial): W.

How old are you? 55-64.

What was your first thought upon seeing yourself with a bald head? Hate it.

Please rate the following statement: "A woman's hair is her crown and glory": 1 = Strongly Agree, 2 = Generally Agree, 3 = Somewhat Disagree, 4 = Strongly Disagree, 5 = I am not sure/Not Applicable: 2 =Generally Agree.

Do you think if you had alopecia, hair loss, it would change the way you see yourself and live your life? Yes.

If you're in a relationship, would your significant other understand and accept you with hair loss? Would there be a change in the way your partner would see or treat you? Yes, I believe he would.

Prior to seeing this image of yourself, have you ever thought about what if you lost your hair? Yes.

Have you ever had an opinion, positive or negative, about seeing a woman with hair loss? Yes.

If so, to the above question, please explain: Hate it.

Would you be willing to share your photo or video screenshot of your bald head filter? No.

If you had to pick between a beautiful head of healthy hair or your dream career, which would be more important to you? Why? Oprah, when she had her show.

Would you like to add or share any additional information and thoughts to this survey? No.

* * *

Respondent #4

Is it OK to use your name, or any identifying information, in print? Yes, it is OK.

First name (or initial): Karliece.

Last name (or initial): A.

How old are you? 45-54.

What was your first thought upon seeing yourself with a bald head? It brought back old memories.

Please rate the following statement: "A woman's hair is her crown and glory": 1 = Strongly Agree, 2 = Generally Agree, 3 = Somewhat Disagree, 4 = Strongly Disagree, 5 = I am not sure/Not Applicable: 2 = Generally Agree.

Do you think if you had alopecia, hair loss, it would change the way you see yourself and live your life? Yes, it would.

If you're in a relationship, would your significant other understand and accept you with hair loss? Would there be a change in the way your partner would see or treat you? My husband would accept me and love me the same.

Prior to seeing this image of yourself, have you ever thought about what if you lost your hair? Yes.

Have you ever had an opinion, positive or negative, about seeing a woman with hair loss? Yes.

If so, to the above question, please explain: Seeing a woman with hair loss, I think to myself it may be Cancer.

Would you be willing to share your photo or video screenshot of your bald head filter? Yes.

If you had to pick between a beautiful head of healthy hair or

your dream career, which would be more important to you? Why? Dream career. I think a dream career is more important in my case. Because with all the hair replacement treatments out there, I could easily get help with hair.

Would you like to add or share any additional information and thoughts to this survey? Yes, I have been bald before. I was 8 years old. I had a baseball accident. Skull fracture, I almost died. However, for the life-saving surgery, I needed to be shaved bald. It was a very traumatic experience at such a young age. I remember looking in the mirror thinking my hair would never grow back. Of course, it did, but the process was slow and brutal. Kids were very cruel. As well as some adults accusing my parents of cutting my hair off.

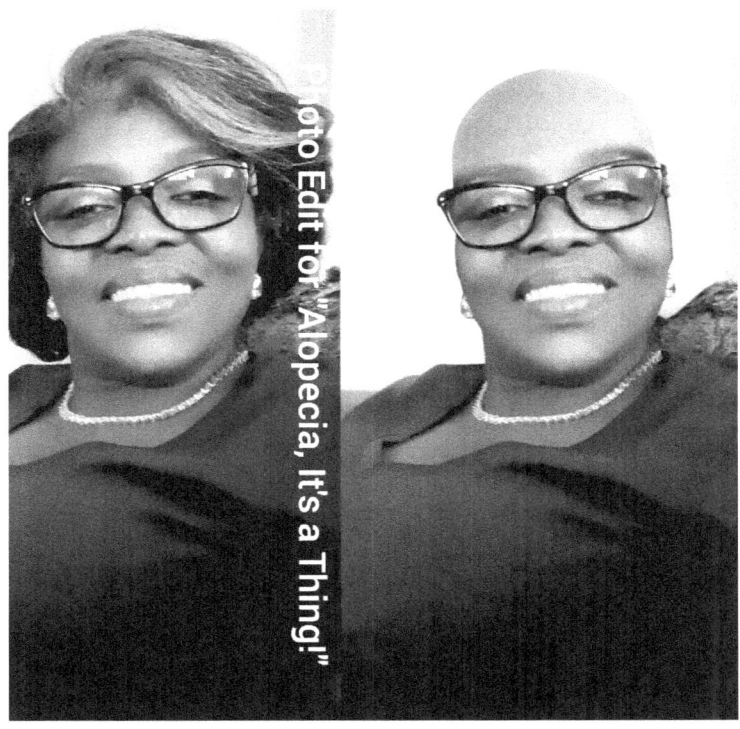

Karliece "PhotoShopped" Photo to Replicate Bald Head

Respondent #5

Is it OK to use your name, or any identifying information, in print? Yes, it is OK.

First name (or initial) Cavisha.

Last name (or initial) W.

How old are you? 45-54.

What was your first thought upon seeing yourself with a bald head? Shocking.

Please rate the following statement: "A woman's hair is her crown and glory": 1 = Strongly Agree, 2 = Generally Agree, 3 = Somewhat Disagree, 4 = Strongly Disagree, 5 = I am not sure/Not Applicable: 1 = Strongly Agree.

Do you think if you had alopecia, hair loss, it would change the way you see yourself and live your life? Would make me self-conscious.

If you're in a relationship, would your significant other understand and accept you with hair loss? Would there be a change in the way your partner would see or treat you? N/A.

Prior to seeing this image of yourself, have you ever thought about what if you lost your hair? No.

Have you ever had an opinion "positive or negative" about seeing a woman with hair loss? No.

If so, to the above question, please explain. N/A.

Would you be willing to share your photo or video screenshot of your bald head filter? No.

If you had to pick between a beautiful head of healthy hair or your dream career, which would be more important to

you? Why? Dream career. I can buy a wig.

Would you like to add/share any additional information or thoughts to this survey? No.

* * *

Respondent #6

Is it OK to use your name, or any identifying information, in print? Yes, it is OK.

First name (or initial): Aubree.

Last name (or initial): M.

How old are you? 35-44.

What was your first thought upon seeing yourself with a bald head? I'm cute!

Please rate the following statement: "A woman's hair is her crown and glory": 1 = Strongly Agree, 2 = Generally Agree, 3 = Somewhat Disagree, 4 = Strongly Disagree, 5 = I am not sure/Not Applicable: 1 = Strongly Agree.

Do you think if you had alopecia, hair loss, it would change the way you see yourself and live your life? It would hurt at first, but then I'd get some great wigs.

If you're in a relationship, would your significant other understand and accept you with hair loss? Would there be a change in the way your partner would see or treat you? Nope, he told me to cut my hair 'cause sometimes I complain about styling it.

Prior to seeing this image of yourself, have you ever thought about what if you lost your hair? Yes.

Have you ever had an opinion "positive or negative" about seeing a woman with hair loss? Yes.

If so, to the above question, please explain: As African-American women, we need to learn how to better take care of our hair.

Would you be willing to share your photo or video screenshot of your bald head filter? Yes.

If you had to pick between a beautiful head of healthy hair or your dream career, which would be more important to you? Why? My dream career.

Would you like to add or share any additional information and thoughts to this survey? No.

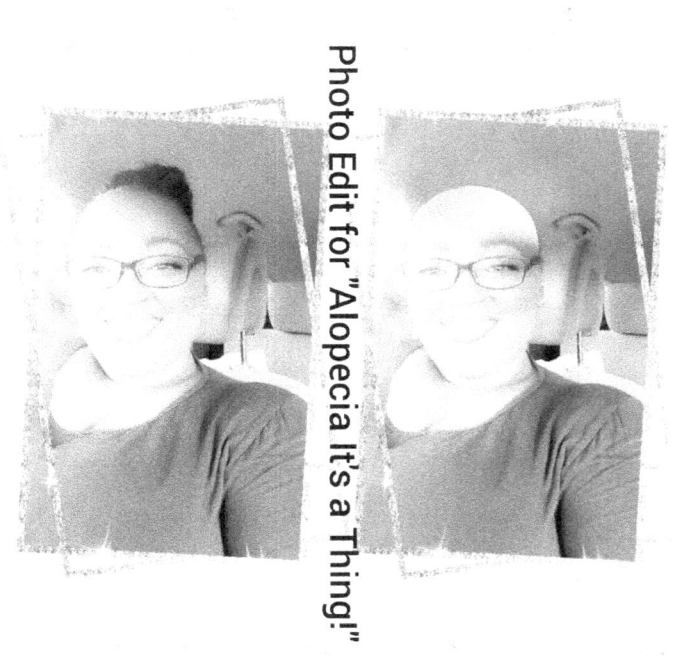

Photo Edit for "Alopecia It's a Thing!"

Aubree "PhotoShopped" Photo to Replicate Bald Head

As I have never been one to ask anyone to do something I am unwilling to do, I decided to participate in the Social Experiment. Below are my before and edited after photos and the answers to the survey. I encourage everyone to try it for themselves. Not to poke fun at, or as a joke but to see what if any feelings it may elicit.

Respondent # 7

Is it OK to use your name, or any identifying information, in print? Yes, it is OK.

First name (or initial): Stephanie.

Last name (or initial): A.

How old are you? 45-54.

What was your first thought upon seeing yourself with a bald head? WOW, was the first reaction that came to mind. Then my jaw dropped, I still saw me. The difference in the picture is definitely visible and profound.

Please rate the following statement: "A woman's hair is her crown and glory": 1 = Strongly Agree, 2 = Generally Agree, 3 = Somewhat Disagree, 4 = Strongly Disagree, 5 = I am not sure/Not Applicable: 1 = Strongly Agree

Do you think if you had alopecia, hair loss, it would change the way you see yourself and live your life? I think it might. Though I accessorize in hair every day, I believe, it may feel different to need to wear it every day as opposed to want to wear it every day.

If you're in a relationship, would your significant other understand and accept you with hair loss? Would there be a change in the way your partner would see or treat you? My husband would accept me. There would be no change.

Prior to seeing this image of yourself, have you ever thought about what if you lost your hair? Yes.

Have you ever had an opinion, positive or negative, about seeing a woman with hair loss? Yes.

If so, to the above question, please explain: I believe a woman is beautiful with or without hair. However, what she chooses to do about it is personal. She shouldn't be made to feel less than.

Would you be willing to share your photo or video screenshot of your bald head filter? Yes.

If you had to pick between a beautiful head of healthy hair or your dream career, which would be more important to you? Why? A dream career, I would just add to my wig collection!

Would you like to add or share any additional information and thoughts to this survey? Yes, I just wanted to use this opportunity to start the discussion about hair loss awareness. I pray this helps to bring light to a subject that most people feel is too painful to discuss.

Thanks to all of you who participated in both surveys!!! Abundant Blessings!

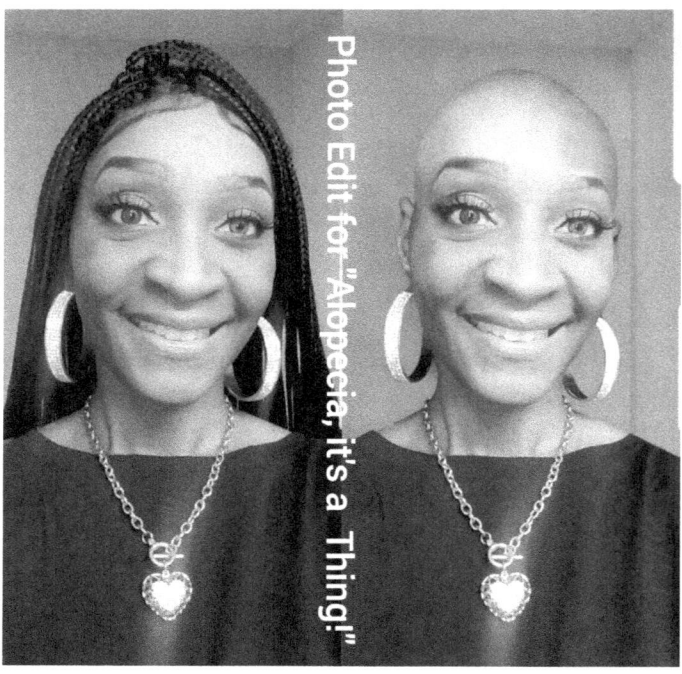

Stephanie Anderson "PhotoShopped" photo to Replicate Bald Head

No Apps/ No Filters

We had the opportunity to learn about celebrities with alopecia. View other celebrities through the eyes of a "balderized" filter. Hear from a small sampling of women without hair loss who see themselves through a "bald" app.

The following pages contain the unedited and actual responses of the survey participants about hair loss from those who have alopecia.

Respondent #1

Is it OK to use your name, or any identifying information, in print? No, it is not OK.

Approximately, when did you first notice hair loss or thinning hair? 3/30/1993

How old are you? 55-64

Are you male or female? Female

Have you been diagnosed with Alopecia? (Alopecia Areata, Alopecia Totalis, Alopecia Universalis, CCCA, Traction Alopecia, Telogen Efflu-vium, Trichotillomania, etc.) If so, which one? It's hormonal, Female Pattern Baldness (Androgenetic Alopecia).

Please rate the following statement: "A woman's hair is her crown and glory": 1 = Strongly Agree, 2 = Generally Agree, 3 = Somewhat Disagree, 4 = Strongly Disagree, 5 = I am not sure/Not Applicable: 1 = Strongly Agree.

How would you explain having alopecia, has it changed the way you see and live your life? I plan my day according to how I can style or manage my wig, to adjust to my daily activities.

What do you see, when you look in the mirror? I really hate to look, or take pictures.

If you're in a relationship, does your significant other understand and accept your diagnosis? Has there been a change in the way your partner sees or treats you? I don't worry about the current, I would on any future partners.

Do you feel self-conscious or ever noticed or caught others looking at your hair? Yes.

In social settings, having alopecia, does it keep you from going out or being around others? If so, please explain: Yes, if they would detect it was a wig or weave.

Is it your understanding that alopecia is an autoimmune disease? Yes.

Do you feel there is any hope, or cure for your hair loss or thinning? Yes.

If you are single, widowed or divorced, will having alopecia have an impact on dating, or being around the opposite sex? If so, please explain. Would that person reject or wonder why.

Do you feel Alopecia has affected your femininity? If so, please explain. Yes, there is nothing that can affect you like the loss of your crowning glory.

In a society where many are judged by their appearance, do you feel like a fake, or less authentic, by wearing a weave, wig, toupee, or extensions? If so, please explain: I feel as if I must, I would look sick without it

If wearing any of the above, is there a fear of them blowing away or being exposed? If so, please explain: Yes always; while walking if the wind blows, or someone just yanks it off.

Initially, when you started losing your hair, did you think it was temporary? Do you feel you were prepared for your new normal. If so, please explain: I thought after a few months it would return, my hair.

How likely have you or would you share your diagnosis of Alopecia with others. 1 = Will NEVER Share, 5 = Definitely will or have Shared: 1= I will never share

If you had to pick between a beautiful head of healthy hair or your dream career, which would be more important to you? Why? This is too close to call.

Would you like to add or share any additional information and thoughts to this survey? No.

Respondent #2

Is it OK to use your name, or any identifying information, in print? Yes, it is OK.

First name (or initial) G.

Last name (or initial) Carter.

Approximately, when did you first notice hair loss or thinning hair? 1/1/1982.

How old are you? 45-54.

Are you male or female? Female

Have you been diagnosed with Alopecia? (Alopecia Areata, Alope-cia Totalis, Alopecia Universalis, CCCA, Traction Alopecia, Telogen Effluvium, Trichotillomania, etc.) If so, which Androgenetic alopecia.

Please rate the following statement: "A woman's hair is her crown and glory": 1 = Strongly Agree, 2 = Generally Agree, 3 = Somewhat Disagree, 4 = Strongly Disagree, 5 = I am not sure/Not Applicable 1 = Strongly Agree.

How would you explain having alopecia, has it changed the way you see and live your life? It has changed my life in profoundly negative ways. It eroded my self-confidence and self-esteem. Alopecia robbed me of participating in many activities and has caused me many embarrassing moments.

What do you see, when you look in the mirror? Without my wig on, I see myself as a very unattractive, aged, depressed woman.

If you're in a relationship, does your significant other understand and accept your diagnosis? Has there been a change in the way your partner sees or treats you? I am married to a very accepting, loving, and supportive man.

Do you feel self-conscious or ever noticed or caught others looking at your hair? Yes

In social settings, having alopecia, does it keep you from going out or being around others? If so, please explain: Depending on the social event, yes, it has kept me from going. For example, I do not go on speed boats or water skiing, activities I used to enjoy a lot. I also was the only person in our large family to not dive off a boat in the ocean due to the fear of my wig falling off in the water.

Is it your understanding that alopecia is an autoimmune disease? No.

Do you feel there is any hope, or cure for your hair loss or thinning? No.

If you are single, widowed or divorced, will having alopecia have an impact on dating, or being around the opposite sex? If so, please explain: If my husband dies before I do, which I hope he doesn't, I don't feel like I could date, nor would I would want to for many reasons; but having hair loss would factor into my decision.

Do you feel Alopecia has affected your femininity? Yes, very much so. Women take pride in their hair and usually like to feel beautiful with attractive hairstyles. I have lost that feeling and long for it every day.

In a society where many are judged by their appearance, do you feel like a fake, or less authentic, by wearing a weave, wig, toupee, or extensions? If so, please explain: I don't feel like a fake, but I do feel insecure sometimes. I have finally accepted people's compliments about my "hair"—it's nice to know people think it looks natural and not a wig.

If wearing any of the above, is there a fear of them blowing away or being exposed? If so, please explain: Yes, even though I wear a head band to secure my wig, if it's too windy or I'm in a crowd, or dancing, I worry that it might come off, or someone may see me adjusting it to my head.

Initially, when you started losing your hair, did you think it was temporary? Do you feel you were prepared for your new normal. If so, please explain: Since I was a young teen when I first noticed it, I did think it was temporary and maybe just my hormones. Actually, when I got older, my hair did get thicker but I was always kind of think on the top near my forehead. After my first child, my hair really changed and got very thin and unhealthy looking. After my second child, it really got bad and never recovered.

How likely have you or would you share your diagnosis of Alopecia with others. 1 = Will NEVER Share, 5 = Definitely will or have Share: 4= I may share

If you had to pick between a beautiful head of healthy hair or your dream career, which would be more important to you? Why? A beautiful head of healthy hair, I could live the life I want to.

Would you like to add or share any additional information and thoughts to this survey? Yes, I appreciate this survey, but it stirred up a lot of emotions. I've never been asked these personal questions. I know things could be a lot worse for me, but my hair loss has caused me great pain for many, many years.

Respondent #3

Is it OK to use your name, or any identifying information, in print? No, it is not.

First name (or initial): N/A

Last name (or initial): N/A

Approximately, when did you first notice hair loss or thinning hair? January 2006

How old are you? 45-54

Are you male or female? Female

Have you been diagnosed with Alopecia? (Alopecia Areata, Alopecia Totalis, Alopecia Universalis, CCCA, Traction Alopecia, Telogen Ef-fluvium, Trichotillomania, etc.) If so, which: Scarring Alopecia (CCCA), Traction Alopecia, Female Pattern Hair Loss,

Please rate the following statement: "A woman's hair is her crown and glory": 1 = Strongly Agree, 2 = Generally Agree, 3 = Somewhat Disagree, 4 = Strongly Disagree, 5 = I am not sure/Not Applicable: 1 = Strongly Agree.

How would you explain having alopecia, has it changed the way you see and live your life? Gradually losing my hair over the years has been one of my best-kept secrets. Thankfully, a lot of women without hair loss wear wigs, weaves, and extensions nowadays. It feels exhausting trying to keep things under the radar. Never wanting to draw attention to myself.

What do you see, when you look in the mirror? A beautiful, vibrant woman who is losing her hair.

If you're in a relationship, does your significant other understand and accept your diagnosis? Has there been a change in the way your partner sees or treats you.? My husband is my best friend. He is aware of the situation but doesn't want to "see" it firsthand.

Do you feel self-conscious or ever noticed or caught others looking at your hair? I feel self-conscious. Mainly, the stares are from people admiring my hairstyles, wig or weave, and asking me for my stylist's contact information.

In social settings, having alopecia, does it keep you from going out or being around others? If so, please explain: No, I am still very social. My job requires me to be out and about all the time. I am aware of my appearance, hair, at all times.

Is it your understanding that alopecia is an autoimmune disease? Yes.

Do you feel there is any hope, or cure for your hair loss or thinning? Yes, in the distant future.

If you are single, widowed or divorced, will having alopecia have an impact on dating, or being around the opposite sex? If so, please explain: N/A.

Do you feel Alopecia has affected your femininity? Yes and No. Yes, because I am locked into wearing artificial hair. No, because when I am wearing hair, I still feel feminine and beautiful.

In a society where many are judged by their appearance, do you feel like a fake. or less authentic, by wearing a weave, wig, toupee, or extensions? If so, please explain: Yes, in some ways I do. Before wigs, weaves, and extensions became popular, it was a taboo to wear anything other than your own hair. Now, even while losing my hair, I blend in.

If wearing any of the above, is there a fear of them blowing away or being exposed? If so, please explain: Yes, only if I don't tape it down or secure it properly.

Initially, when you started losing your hair, did you think it was temporary? Do you feel you were prepared for your new normal. If so, please explain: Yes, I thought it was temporary. I was not prepared.

How likely have you or would you share your diagnosis of Alopecia with others. 1 = Will NEVER Share, 5 = Definitely will or have Shared: 1=I will NEVER share.

If you had to pick between a beautiful head of healthy hair or your dream career, which would be more important to you? Why? My dream career, I am doing what I LOVE currently. As long as I can look good wearing artificial hair, I feel good about myself.

Would you like to add or share any additional information and thoughts to this survey? No, just want to say thank you, Ms. Anderson, for the opportunity to share my feelings. Losing your hair is so personal. It was therapeutic to talk about it, even anonymously.

Respondent #4

Is it OK to use your name, or any identifying information, in print? Yes, it is OK.

First name (or initial) M.

Last name (or initial) Herron.

Approximately, when did you first notice hair loss or thinning hair? 6/1/2022.

How old are you? 45-54

Are you male or female? Female.

Have you been diagnosed with Alopecia? (Alopecia Areata, Alope-cia Totalis, Alopecia Universalis, CCCA, Traction Alopecia, Telogen Effluvium, Trichotillomania, etc.) If so, which: Alopecia Areata

Please rate the following statement: "A woman's hair is her crown and glory": 1 = Strongly Agree, 2 = Generally Agree, 3 = Somewhat Disagree, 4 = Strongly Disagree, 5 = I am not sure/Not Applicable: 2 = Generally Agree

How would you explain having alopecia, has it changed the way you see and live your life? It's humbled me tremendously.

What do you see, when you look in the mirror? A woman with ugly bald spots, but I see a beautiful woman underneath.

If you're in a relationship, does your significant other understand and accept your diagnosis? Has there been a change the way your partner sees or treats you? Single, however I see how men view me differently, now that I'm bald with spots.

Do you feel self- conscious or ever noticed or caught others looking at your hair? Yes.

In social settings, having alopecia, does it keep you from going out or being around others? If so, please explain Yes, because going through menopause, it's hard to cover up my head without suffering hot flashes. But I also don't like being stared at with the bald spots.

Is it your understanding that alopecia is an autoimmune disease? Yes.

Do you feel there is any hope, or cure for your hair loss or thinning? No.

If you are single, widowed or divorced, will having alopecia have an impact on dating, or being around the opposite sex? If so, please explain: Yes, because men can be so shallow when it comes to what they look for in a woman. Nothing about her character, its all about the looks with men.

Do you feel Alopecia has affected your femininity? No, I'm still all woman, inside and out.

In a society where many are judged by their appearance, do you feel like a fake, or less authentic, by wearing a weave, wig, toupee, or extensions? If so, please explain. Not fake, but we shouldn't hide behind those artificial things.

If wearing any of the above, is there a fear of them blowing away or being exposed? If so, please explain. No.

Initially, when you started losing your hair, did you think it was temporary? Do you feel you were prepared for your new normal. If so, please explain: I thought it was temporary, however I see that it possibly isn't. However, I know I can't let it distract me from a beautiful future that God has for me.

How likely have you or would you share your diagnosis of Alopecia with others. 1 = Will NEVER Share, 5 = Definitely will or have shared: 5= Definitely will or have Shared.

If you had to pick between a beautiful head of healthy hair or your dream career, which would be more important to you? Why? Dream career, hair doesn't make me who I am.

Would you like to add or share any additional information and thoughts to this survey? No.

Respondent #5

Is it OK to use your name, or any identifying information, in print? Yes, it is OK.

First name (or initial): T.

Last name (or initial): Daniels.

Approximately, when did you first notice hair loss or thinning hair? 7/18/2015.

How old are you? 45-54.

Are you male or female? Female.

Have you been diagnosed with Alopecia? (Alopecia Areata, Alope-cia Totalis, Alopecia Universalis, CCCA, Traction Alopecia, Telogen Effluvium, Trichotillomania, etc.) If so, which: CCCA.

Please rate the following statement: "A woman's hair is her crown and glory": 1 = Strongly Agree, 2 = Generally Agree, 3 = Somewhat Disagree, 4 = Strongly Disagree, 5 = I am not sure/Not Applicable: 1 = Strongly Agree.

How would you explain having alopecia, has it changed the way you see and live your life? It makes you feel uncomfortable about the way you look, but once I cut my hair low, I began to see my beauty again. Especially when other women started wearing short cuts and wigs.

What do you see, when you look in the mirror? A beautiful balding woman. Before, I was depressed to see my hair loss.

If you're in a relationship, does your significant other understand and accept your diagnosis? Has there been a change the way your partner sees or treats you? N/A.

Do you feel self-conscious or ever noticed or caught others looking at your hair? Yes.

In social settings, having alopecia, does it keep you from going out or being around others? If so, please explain: If I wore a wig, I wondered if others could tell; and with the short cut, I hoped I wasn't mistaken for a man.

Is it your understanding that alopecia is an autoimmune disease? No.

Do you feel there is any hope, or cure for your hair loss or thinning? No.

If you are single, widowed or divorced, will having alopecia have an impact on dating, or being around the opposite sex? If so, please explain: I don't think so because I wear my short hair and many men know women wear wigs and different styles now. I'm just honest and allow the opposite sex to see me with my wig, and without a wig.

Do you feel Alopecia has affected your femininity? No, not at all.

In a society where many are judged by their appearance, do you feel like a fake, or less authentic, by wearing a weave, wig, toupee, or extensions? If so, please explain: No, I don't because it's trending now and everyone wears their hair with at least one of these types of styles.

If wearing any of the above, is there a fear of them blowing away or being exposed? If so, please explain: Sometimes.

Initially, when you started losing your hair, did you think it was temporary? Do you feel you were prepared for your new normal. If so, please explain: I felt it was going to be the new normal and had to figure out how to have hair to wear once it was gone.

How likely have you or would you share your diagnosis of Alopecia with others. 1 = Will NEVER Share, 5 = Definitely will or have Shared: 4=I may share

If you had a choice to pick a beautiful head of healthy hair or your dream career, which would be more important to you? Why? A beautiful head of hair. Because at some point that career will end. But you could keep your hair forever if it stays healthy.

Would you like to add or share any additional information and thoughts to this survey? No.

Respondent #6

Is it OK to use your name, or any identifying information, in print? No, it's not OK.

First name (or initial): N/A.

Last name (or initial): N/A.

Approximately, when did you first notice hair loss or thinning hair? 12/12/2000.

How old are you? 65+.

Are you male or female? Female.

Have you been diagnosed with Alopecia? (Alopecia Areata, Alope-cia Totalis, Alopecia Universalis, CCCA, Traction Alopecia, Telogen Effluvium, Trichotillomania, etc.) If so, which: Alopecia.

Please rate the following statement: "A woman's hair is her crown and glory": 1 = Strongly Agree, 2 = Generally Agree, 3 = Somewhat Disagree, 4 = Strongly Disagree, 5 = I am not sure/Not Applicable: 1 = Strongly Agree

How would you explain having alopecia, has it changed the way you see and live your life? Yes, it totally changed my life.

What do you see, when you look in the mirror? Wish that I didn't lose my hair.

If you're in a relationship, does your significant other understand and accept your diagnosis? Has there been a change the way your partner sees or treats you? He completely understands.

Do you feel self-conscious or ever noticed or caught others looking at your hair? Yes.

In social settings, having alopecia, does it keep you from going out or being around others? If so, please explain Sometimes, if my hair, wig, needs maintenance.

Is it your understanding that alopecia is an autoimmune disease? No.

Do you feel there is any hope, or cure for your hair loss or thinning? No.

If you are single, widowed or divorced, will having alopecia have an impact on dating, or being around the opposite sex? If so, please explain. No.

Do you feel Alopecia has affected your femininity? No.

In a society where many are judged by their appearance, do you feel like a fake, or less authentic, by wearing a weave, wig, toupee, or extensions? If so, please explain: No, a lot of people wear fake hair.

If wearing any of the above, is there a fear of them blowing away or being exposed? If so, please explain: No.

Initially, when you started losing your hair, did you think it was temporary? Do you feel you were prepared for your new normal. If so, please explain: No, I was in shock.

How likely have you or would you share your diagnosis of Alopecia with others. 1 = Will NEVER Share, 5 = Definitely will or have Shared: 5 = I Definitely will or have shared.

If you had to pick between a beautiful head of healthy hair or your dream career, which would be more important to you? Why? My hair, because it's for life.

Would you like to add or share any additional information and thoughts to this survey? No.

Respondent #7

Is it OK to use your name, or any identifying information, in print? Yes, it is OK.

First name (or initial): T.

Last name (or initial): Douglas.

Approximately, when did you first notice hair loss or thinning hair? 6/1/2001.

How old are you? 55-64.

Are you male or female? Female.

Have you been diagnosed with Alopecia? (Alopecia Areata, Alope-cia Totalis, Alopecia Universalis, CCCA, Traction Alopecia, Telogen Effluvium, Trichotillomania, etc.) If so, which: Yes.

Please rate the following statement: "A woman's hair is her crown and glory": 1 = Strongly Agree, 2 = Generally Agree, 3 = Somewhat Disagree, 4 = Strongly Disagree, 5 = I am not sure/Not Applicable: 1 = Strongly Agree.

How would you explain having alopecia, has it changed the way you see and live your life? Absolutely. I will always have to wear weaves or wigs.

What do you see, when you look in the mirror? I don't like to look at my hair in the mirror. When I style my extensions, I pray for a miracle...to be able to style my own hair.

If you're in a relationship, does your significant other understand and accept your diagnosis? Has there been a change the way your partner sees or treats you? Hair loss is one of the reasons why I'm not in a relationship. I don't feel beautiful because I don't have hair.

Do you feel self-conscious or ever noticed or caught others looking at your hair? Yes.

In social settings, having alopecia, does it keep you from going out or being around others? If so, please explain Yes, I'm always thinking about someone pulling off my wig just to get a laugh.

Is it your understanding that alopecia is an autoimmune disease? No.

Do you feel there is any hope, or cure for your hair loss or thinning? No.

If you are single, widowed or divorced, will having alopecia have an impact on dating, or being around the opposite sex? If so, please explain Yes, it does. Hair is another element that adds to our beauty. Bald spots are not attractive on me.

Do you feel Alopecia has affected your femininity? No.

In a society where many are judged by their appearance, do you feel like a fake, or less authentic, by wearing a weave, wig, toupee, or extensions? If so, please explain: Yes. Having to alter your appearance by any type of augmentation can be viewed as fake. The end result is others will question why you're trying to be something else.

If wearing any of the above, is there a fear of them blowing away or being exposed? If so, please explain: Yes. I went to Chicago and because it's the windy city, I had to take extra precautions.

Initially, when you started losing your hair, did you think it was temporary? Do you feel you were prepared for your new normal. If so, please explain: Yes. I thought it was temporary. Serving in the military and living in different countries, I thought the harsh water was causing my hair loss. I believed at some point it would grow back. No, I was not prepared to live my prime years with hair loss.

How likely have you or would you share your diagnosis of Alopecia with others. 1 = Will NEVER Share, 5 = Definitely will or have Shared: 3 =I am unsure.

If you had to pick between a beautiful head of healthy hair or your dream career, which would be more important to you? Why? A healthy head of hair. If I'm happy, I can make any career a dream.

Would you like to add or share any additional information and thoughts to this survey? No.

Respondent #8

Is it OK to use your name, or any identifying information, in print? Yes, it is OK.

First name (or initial): B.

Last name (or initial): Rankins.

Approximately, when did you first notice hair loss or thinning hair? 11/7/2020.

How old are you? 55-64.

Are you male or female? Female.

Have you been diagnosed with Alopecia? (Alopecia Areata, Alope-cia Totalis, Alopecia Universalis, CCCA, Traction Alopecia, Telogen Effluvium, Trichotillomania, etc.) If so, which: Vitiligo

Please rate the following statement: "A woman's hair is her crown and glory": 1 = Strongly Agree, 2 = Generally Agree, 3 = Somewhat Disagree, 4 = Strongly Disagree, 5 = I am not sure/Not Applicable: 2 = Generally Agree.

How would you explain having alopecia, has it changed the way you see and live your life? N/A; however, thin hair with vitiligo on your scalp looks like a fire victim.

What do you see, when you look in the mirror? Disfigurement.

If you're in a relationship, does your significant other understand and accept your diagnosis? Has there been a change the way your partner sees or treats you? Yes, he understands; grateful for life.

Do you feel self-conscious or ever noticed or caught others looking at your hair? No.

In social settings, having alopecia, does it keep you from going out or being around others? If so, please explain: N/A, but I do wear wigs.

Is it your understanding that alopecia is an autoimmune disease? Yes.

Do you feel there is any hope, or cure for your hair loss or thinning? No.

If you are single, widowed or divorced, will having alopecia have an impact on dating, or being around the opposite sex? If so, please explain Married for 40 years, and very conscientious of how I look.

Do you feel Alopecia has affected your femininity? No.

In a society where many are judged by their appearance, do you feel like a fake, or less authentic, by wearing a weave, wig, toupee, or extensions? If so, please explain: No.

If wearing any of the above, is there a fear of them blowing away or being exposed? If so, please explain: Yes.

Initially, when you started losing your hair, did you think it was temporary? Do you feel you were prepared for your new normal. If so, please explain: No. Never been accepted living with it.

How likely have you or would you share your diagnosis of Alopecia with others. 1 = Will NEVER Share, 5 = Definitely will or have Shared: 4 = I may share

If you had to pick between a beautiful head of healthy hair or your dream career, which would be more important to you? Why? At this point in my life, healthy hair. I'm retired; love salt and pepper hair, being my best at my age. Looking good, feeling good.

Would you like to add or share any additional information and thoughts to this survey? Yes, not everyone wants to cover their grey. There are those that want long, silky, natural hair replacement choices.

Respondent #9

Is it OK to use your name, or any identifying information, in print? No, it is not.

Approximately, when did you first notice hair loss or thinning hair? 10/14/1980.

How old are you? 35-44.

Are you male or female? Female.

Have you been diagnosed with Alopecia? Alopecia Areata, Alope-cia Totalis, Alopecia Universalis, CCCA, Traction Alopecia, Telogen Effluvium, Trichotillomania, etc. If so, which: No.

Please rate the following statement: "A woman's hair is her crown and glory": 1 = Strongly Agree, 2 = Generally Agree, 3 = Somewhat Disagree, 4 = Strongly Disagree, 5 = I am not sure/Not Applicable: 1 = Strongly Agree

How would you explain having alopecia, has it changed the way you see and live your life? N/A.

What do you see, when you look in the mirror? A woman who wishes she had her own full head of hair instead of wearing a wig.

If you're in a relationship, does your significant other understand and accept your diagnosis? Has there been a change the way your partner sees or treats you? We have not had this discussion.

Do you feel self-conscious or ever noticed or caught others looking at your hair? Yes.

In social settings, having alopecia, does it keep you from going out or being around others? If so, please explain: No experience with alopecia.

Is it your understanding that alopecia is an autoimmune disease? Yes.

Do you feel there is any hope, or cure for your hair loss or thinning? Yes.

If you are single, widowed or divorced, will having alopecia have an impact on dating, or being around the opposite sex? If so, please explain: No.

Do you feel Alopecia has affected your femininity? No.

In a society where many are judged by their appearance, do you feel like a fake, or less authentic, by wearing a weave, wig, toupee, or extensions? If so, please explain: No.

If wearing any of the above, is there a fear of them blowing away or being exposed? If so, please explain: No.

Initially, when you started losing your hair, did you think it was temporary? Do you feel you were prepared for your new normal. If so, please explain: No.

How likely have you or would you share your diagnosis of Alopecia with others. 1 = Will NEVER Share, 5 = Definitely will or have Share: 5 = Definitely will or have Share

If you had to pick between a beautiful head of healthy hair or your dream career, which would be more important to you? Why? Hair, because beautiful, healthy hair enhances your appearance.

Would you like to add or share any additional information and thoughts to this survey? No.

Respondent #10

Is it OK to use your name, or any identifying information, in print? Yes, it is OK.

First name (or initial): Toria.

Last name (or initial): B.

Approximately, when did you first notice hair loss or thinning hair? 1/2/2019.

How old are you? 18-24.

Are you male or female? Female

Have you been diagnosed with Alopecia? (Alopecia Areata, Alope-cia Totalis, Alopecia Universalis, CCCA, Traction Alopecia, Telogen Effluvium, Trichotillomania, etc.) If so, which: No

Please rate the following statement: "A woman's hair is her crown and glory": 1 = Strongly Agree, 2 = Generally Agree, 3 = Somewhat Disagree, 4 = Strongly Disagree, 5 = I am not sure/Not Applicable: 1 = Strongly Agree

How would you explain having alopecia, has it changed the way you see and live your life? Most times it gives a low self esteem; especially when you see other females with healthy hair.

What do you see, when you look in the mirror? A beautiful woman.

If you're in a relationship, does your significant other understand and accept your diagnosis? Has there been a change the way your partner sees or treats you? No.

Do you feel self-conscious or ever noticed or caught others looking at your hair? Yes.

In social settings, having alopecia, does it keep you from going out or being around others? If so, please explain No, it does not.

Is it your understanding that alopecia is an autoimmune disease? No.

Do you feel there is any hope, or cure for your hair loss or thinning? Yes.

If you are single, widowed or divorced, will having alopecia have an impact on dating, or being around the opposite sex? If so, please explain: No.

Do you feel Alopecia has affected your femininity? No.

In a society where many are judged by their appearance, do you feel like a fake, or less authentic, by wearing a weave, wig, toupee, or extensions? If so, please explain: No I don't, I wear very nice wigs.

If wearing any of the above, is there a fear of them blowing away or being exposed? If so, please explain: Yes, most times I'm scared when there's heavy breeze. I tend to hold on tight to my wig.

Initially, when you started losing your hair, did you think it was temporary? Do you feel you were prepared for your new normal. If so, please explain: Yes, I had my hair cut.

How likely have you or would you share your diagnosis of Alopecia with others. 1 = Will NEVER Share, 5 = Definitely will or have Shared: 5=Definitely will or have Shared.

If you had to pick between a beautiful head of healthy hair or your dream career, which would be more important to you? Why? My dream career. Who I want to be matters to me, it is not really about how others see me, but about how I see myself.

Would you like to add or share any additional information and thoughts to this survey? No.

Respondent #11

Is it OK to use your name, or any identifying information, in print? Yes, it is OK.

First name (or initial): B.

Last name (or initial): L.

Approximately, when did you first notice hair loss or thinning hair? 1/31/2013.

How old are you? 55-64.

Are you male or female? Female.

Have you been diagnosed with Alopecia? (Alopecia Areata, Alope-cia Totalis, Alopecia Universalis, CCCA, Traction Alopecia, Telogen Effluvium, Trichotillomania, etc.) If so, which: No.

Please rate the following statement: "A woman's hair is her crown and glory": 1 = Strongly Agree, 2 = Generally Agree, 3 = Somewhat Disagree, 4 = Strongly Disagree, 5 = I am not sure/Not Applicable: 1 = Strongly Agree.

How would you explain having alopecia, has it changed the way you see and live your life? No alopecia, but thinning hair in the crown of my head.

What do you see when you look in the mirror? I still see a beautiful woman, only wishing that I had thicker hair. When I think of others that don't even have as much hair as I have, I have a feeling of gratitude.

If you're in a relationship, does your significant other understand and accept your diagnosis? Has there been a change the way your partner sees or treats you? There has been the acceptance and no remarks made to the thinning of hair.

Do you feel self-conscious or ever noticed or caught others looking at your hair? Yes.

In social settings, having alopecia, does it keep you from going out or being around others? If so, please explain: Do not normally let thinning hair keep me from social settings.

Is it your understanding that alopecia is an autoimmune disease? No.

Do you feel there is any hope, or cure for your hair loss or thinning? Yes.

If you are single, widowed or divorced, will having alopecia have an impact on dating, or being around the opposite sex? If so, please explain: N/A.

Do you feel Alopecia has affected your femininity? Thinning hair has not affected my femininity. Thank goodness for short hair and shaved heads for women becoming popular.

In a society where many are judged by their appearance, do you feel like a fake, or less authentic, by wearing a weave, wig, toupee, or extensions? If so, please explain: The popularity of wigs is so acceptable, I don't believe one feels fake by wearing them

If wearing any of the above, is there a fear of them blowing away or being exposed? If so, please explain: There is always that chance, I personally prefer no wigs unless for fun. I don't think there is a lot of worry about being exposed if revealed one is wearing one

Initially, when you started losing your hair, did you think it was temporary? Do you feel you were prepared for your new normal. If so, please explain: I thought it may be temporary, but also believe age is a factor and didn't expect to keep the thickness of my hair like in my youth. Also, hearing that women and men have hair loss, helps a bit with acceptance.

How likely have you, or would you, share your diagnosis of Alopecia with others. 1 = Will NEVER Share, 5 = Definitely will or have Shared: 5=Definitely will or have Shared.

If you had to pick between a beautiful head of healthy hair or your dream career, which would be more important to you? Why? Maybe the dream career, because you could afford to buy some healthy hair or not.

Would you like to add or share any additional information and thoughts to this survey? Yes, I believe that as we mature there is less concern with hair and more focused on life. With so many styles and types of wigs, hair pieces, etc., there seems to be a greater acceptance among people.

Respondent #12

Is it OK to use your name, or any identifying information, in print? Yes, it is OK.

First name (or initial): M.

Last name (or initial): Hawkins.

Approximately, when did you first notice hair loss or thinning hair? 8/5/2004.

How old are you? 45-54.

Are you male or female? Female.

Have you been diagnosed with Alopecia? (Alopecia Areata, Aope-cia Totalis, Alopecia Universalis, CCCA, Traction Alopecia, Telogen Effluvium, Trichotillomania, etc.) If so, which: Frontal Fibrosing alopecia.

Please rate the following statement: "A woman's hair is her crown and glory": 1 = Strongly Agree, 2 = Generally Agree, 3 = Somewhat Disagree, 4 = Strongly Disagree, 5 = I am not sure/Not Applicable: 1 = Strongly Agree

How would you explain having alopecia, has it changed the way you see and live your life? It's been a huge and humbling change.

What do you see, when you look in the mirror? My hairline receding more every year.

If you're in a relationship, does your significant other understand and accept your diagnosis? Has there been a change the way your partner sees or treats you.? Got divorced and have no desire to even try dating again.

Do you feel self-conscious or ever noticed or caught others looking at your hair? Yes.

In social settings, having alopecia, does it keep you from going out or being around others? If so, please explain: Yes—don't enjoy going out like I used to because I don't feel attractive.

Is it your understanding that alopecia is an autoimmune disease? Yes.

Do you feel there is any hope, or cure for your hair loss or thinning? No.

If you are single, widowed or divorced, will having alopecia have an impact on dating, or being around the opposite sex? If so, please explain: Yes, I used to love to go out and mingle when I felt I looked good—that no longer applies.

Do you feel Alopecia has affected your femininity? Yes—I don't feel attractive

In a society where many are judged by their appearance, do you feel like a fake, or less authentic, by wearing a weave, wig, toupee, or extensions? If so, please explain: No, but wigs are not as comfortable as wearing a baseball cap.

If wearing any of the above, is there a fear of them blowing away or being exposed? If so, please explain: Yes, usually wear a hairband under hat in case it has to come off.

Initially, when you started losing your hair, did you think it was temporary? Do you feel you were prepared for your new normal. If so, please explain: Did not want to accept it for many years.

How likely have you or would you share your diagnosis of Alopecia with others. 1 = Will NEVER Share, 5 = Definitely will or have Shared: 5 = Definitely will or have Shared.

If you had to pick between a beautiful head of healthy hair or your dream career, which would be more important to

you? Why? My hair over career because it was part of who I am identified with.

Would you like to add or share any additional information and thoughts to this survey? No.

Respondent #13

Is it OK to use your name, or any identifying information, in print? Yes, it is OK.

First name (or initial): G.O.

Last name (or initial): Byrd

Approximately, when did you first notice hair loss or thinning hair? 5/1/1986.

How old are you? 65+.

Are you male or female? Female.

Have you been diagnosed with Alopecia? (Alopecia Areata, Alope-cia Totalis, Alopecia Universalis, CCCA, Traction Alopecia, Telogen Effluvium, Trichotillomania, etc.) If so, which: Yes.

Please rate the following statement: "A woman's hair is her crown and glory": 1 = Strongly Agree, 2 = Generally Agree, 3 = Somewhat Disagree, 4 = Strongly Disagree, 5 = I am not sure/Not Applicable: 4 = Strongly Disagree.

How would you explain having alopecia, has it changed the way you see and live your life? Wearing a wig or wrap constantly makes me uncomfortable in settings where natural hair or no hair are the norm. I scuba dive and don't have a wig, I feel comfortable diving in. So, I've stopped diving. Exercising and being active, swimming or bike riding is hot enough in 90+ degree weather with a wig, plus protective gear on head at times.

What do you see, when you look in the mirror? It depends on the day and time, and what mood I'm in.

If you're in a relationship, does your significant other understand and accept your diagnosis? Has there been a change the way your partner sees or treats you? N/A.

Do you feel self-conscious or ever noticed or caught others looking at your hair? No.

In social settings, having alopecia, does it keep you from going out or being around others? If so, please explain: No.

Is it your understanding that alopecia is an autoimmune disease? Yes.

Do you feel there is any hope, or cure for your hair loss or thinning? No.

If you are single, widowed or divorced, will having alopecia have an impact on dating, or being around the opposite sex? If so, please explain: Yes, for sure. Some men do not care for wigs on their partners, so I'd definitely steer clear of a relationship with a man like that.

Do you feel Alopecia has affected your femininity? No, my femininity is intact with or without hair. I do wish that the hair I have that grows around the edges of my face would quit growing. My crown is bald; so if I were a man, I'd either shave it or wear a man's weave to hide my loss of hair.

In a society where many are judged by their appearance, do you feel like a fake, or less authentic, by wearing a weave, wig, toupee, or extensions? If so, please explain: I don't feel like a fake, but I sometimes get tired of always putting something on my head when I go out.

If wearing any of the above, is there a fear of them blowing away or being exposed? If so, please explain: I would absolutely hate it if my wig was forcibly removed from my head, plus that would be assault if it's done by another other than me.

Initially, when you started losing your hair, did you think it was temporary? Do you feel you were prepared for your new normal. If so, please explain: I thought my hair loss was temporary until I saw how smooth my scalp was and reality set in:

my hair was gone forever. I was not prepared, initially. But over the years, I quickly adapted to my hair loss.

How likely have you or would you share your diagnosis of Alopecia with others. 1 = Will NEVER Share, 5 = Definitely will or have Share: 4=May share

If you had to pick between a beautiful head of healthy hair or your dream career, which would be more important to you? Why? I'd choose my dream career because I'd make enough money to be able to afford a wardrobe full of human hair to wear or not. It's my choice to wear a beautiful head of hair or just my beautiful head.

Would you like to add or share any additional information and thoughts to this survey? No.

Respondent #14

Is it OK to use your name, or any identifying information, in print? Yes, it is OK.

First name (or initial) C.

Last name (or initial) Venter.

Approximately, when did you first notice hair loss or thinning hair? 3/1/21.

How old are you? 35-44.

Are you male or female? Female.

Have you been diagnosed with Alopecia? (Alopecia Areata, Alope-cia Totalis, Alopecia Universalis, CCCA, Traction Alopecia, Telogen Effluvium, Trichotillomania, etc.) If so, which: Yes, Alopecia Areata.

Please rate the following statement: "A woman's hair is her crown and glory": 1 = Strongly Agree, 2 = Generally Agree, 3 = Somewhat Disagree, 4 = Strongly Disagree, 5 = I am not sure/Not Applicable: 4 = Strongly Disagree.

How would you explain having alopecia, has it changed the way you see and live your life? Not having hair, freed me from the societies viewpoint that hair is a woman's crown of glory.

What do you see, when you look in the mirror? A beautiful shaped head.

If you're in a relationship, does your significant other understand and accept your diagnosis? Has there been a change the way your partner sees or treats you? I received my family's full support.

Do you feel self-conscious or ever noticed or caught others looking at your hair? Yes.

In social settings, having alopecia, does it keep you from going out or being around others? If so, please explain: No, I'm embracing my baldness.

Is it your understanding that alopecia is an autoimmune disease? Yes.

Do you feel there is any hope, or cure for your hair loss or thinning? Yes.

If you are single, widowed or divorced, will having alopecia have an impact on dating, or being around the opposite sex? If so, please explain: N/A.

Do you feel Alopecia has affected your femininity? Oh yes. It has made me feel more open and now I can focus my attention on other things like swimming for example without having to worry about my hair.

In a society where many are judged by their appearance, do you feel like a fake (or less authentic) by wearing a weave, wig/toupee, or extensions? If so, please explain. I don't have any. Embrace my baldness.

If wearing any of the above, is there a fear of them blowing away or being exposed? If so, please explain. N/A.

Initially, when you started losing your hair, did you think it was temporary? Do you feel you were prepared for your new normal. If so, please explain: Very little info was given by the doctor. I learned everything I know so far from internet searches and support groups.

How likely have you or would you share your diagnosis of Alopecia with others. 1 = Will NEVER Share, 5 = Definitely will or have Shared: 5=Definitely will or have Share.

If you had to pick between a beautiful head of healthy hair or your dream career, which would be more important to

you? Why? Definitely dream career. Hair don't define me.

Would you like to add or share any additional information and thoughts to this survey? No.

Respondent #15

Is it OK to use your name, or any identifying information, in print? Yes, it is OK.

First name (or initial): T.

Last name (or initial): M.

Approximately, when did you first notice hair loss or thinning hair? 8/2/1993.

How old are you? 55-64.

Are you male or female? Female.

Have you been diagnosed with Alopecia? (Alopecia Areata, Alope-cia Totalis, Alopecia Universalis, CCCA, Traction Alopecia, Telogen Effluvium, Trichotillomania, etc.) If so, which: Alopecia Areata.

Please rate the following statement: "A woman's hair is her crown and glory": 1 = Strongly Agree, 2 = Generally Agree, 3 = Somewhat Disagree, 4 = Strongly Disagree, 5 = I am not sure/Not Applicable: 1 = Strongly Agree.

How would you explain having alopecia, has it changed the way you see and live your life? It has affected my self esteem and self image.

What do you see, when you look in the mirror? A work in progress.

If you're in a relationship, does your significant other understand and accept your diagnosis? Has there been a change the way your partner sees or treats you? My spouse and I haven't discussed it.

Do you feel self-conscious or ever noticed or caught others looking at your hair? Yes.

ALOPECIA, IT'S A THING! BREAKING THROUGH THE B.S. (BELIEF SYSTEMS)

In social settings, having alopecia, does it keep you from going out or being around others? If so, please explain: Yes, initially because you didn't feel comfortable with a wig or having alopecia. You thought everyone would know which would make me feel worse.

Is it your understanding that alopecia is an autoimmune disease? Yes.

Do you feel there is any hope, or cure for your hair loss or thinning? Yes.

If you are single, widowed or divorced, will having alopecia have an impact on dating, or being around the opposite sex? If so, please explain: N/A.

Do you feel Alopecia has affected your femininity? Yes, because a female's hair is seen as her crown and glory.

In a society where many are judged by their appearance, do you feel like a fake (or less authentic) by wearing a weave, wig/toupee, or extensions? If so, please explain: I initially did, until I came two terms with alopecia.

If wearing any of the above, is there a fear of them blowing away or being exposed? If so, please explain: Yes, because there's always been that stigma in the media where you see a wig blowing off or partially coming up on the frontal portion.

Initially, when you started losing your hair, did you think it was temporary? Do you feel you were prepared for your new normal. If so, please explain: Yes, because my hair initially came back in before falling out again. No, no one is ever prepared for alopecia.

How likely have you or would you share your diagnosis of Alopecia with others. 1 = Will NEVER Share, 5 = Definitely will or have Share: 5 = Definitely will or have Share

If you had to pick between a beautiful head of healthy hair or your dream career, which would be more important to you? Why? Beautiful head of healthy hair

Would you like to add or share any additional information and thoughts to this survey? No

Respondent #16

Is it OK to use your name, or any identifying information, in print? No, it is not:

First name (or initial): N/A.

Last name (or initial): N/A.

Approximately, when did you first notice hair loss or thinning hair? 12/12/1974.

How old are you? 65+.

Are you male or female? Female.

Have you been diagnosed with Alopecia? (Alopecia Areata, Alope-cia Totalis, Alopecia Universalis, CCCA, Traction Alopecia, Telogen Effluvium, Trichotillomania, etc.) If so, which: No.

Please rate the following statement: "A woman's hair is her crown and glory": 1 = Strongly Agree, 2 = Generally Agree, 3 = Somewhat Disagree, 4 = Strongly Disagree, 5 = I am not sure/Not Applicable: 1 = Strongly Agree.

How would you explain having alopecia, has it changed the way you see and live your life? It makes me feel less feminine.

What do you see, when you look in the mirror? An unattractive woman.

If you're in a relationship, does your significant other understand and accept your diagnosis? Has there been a change the way your partner sees or treats you? He does not know.

Do you feel self-conscious or ever noticed or caught others looking at your hair? Yes.

In social settings, having alopecia, does it keep you from going out or being around others? If so, please explain: No, I wear wigs but never go out without.

Is it your understanding that alopecia is an autoimmune disease? No.

Do you feel there is any hope, or cure for your hair loss or thinning? Yes.

If you are single, widowed or divorced, will having alopecia have an impact on dating, or being around the opposite sex? If so, please explain: Yes, it would inhibit being intimate.

Do you feel Alopecia has affected your femininity? Yes, because hair is what makes a woman feminine.

In a society where many are judged by their appearance, do you feel like a fake, or less authentic, by wearing a weave, wig, toupee, or extensions? If so, please explain: Yes, because I don't have real hair.

If wearing any of the above, is there a fear of them blowing away or being exposed? If so, please explain: Yes, it would embarrass me to be exposed.

Initially, when you started losing your hair, did you think it was temporary? Do you feel you were prepared for your new normal. If so, please explain: No, I was ashamed and felt like a freak.

How likely have you or would you share your diagnosis of Alopecia with others. 1 = Will NEVER Share, 5 = Definitely will or have Shared: 3=Unsure if I would share.

If you had to pick between a beautiful head of healthy hair or your dream career, which would be more important to you? Why? A career because I could then afford the best wigs or a hair transplant.

Would you like to add or share any additional information and thoughts to this survey? No.

* * *

She is more precious than jewels, and nothing you desire can compare with her. Long life is in her right hand; in her left hand are riches and honor. Her ways are ways of pleasantness, and all her paths are peace. *Proverbs 3: 15-17 (ESV)*

ACKNOWLEDGMENTS

Although you write alone, it takes the support of, patience from, and confidence in a lot of people during your journey of writing, especially for a first-time author like me. I am grateful to the following: Jesslyn Hodges and Mary Moore, my sisters, were the ones who let me bounce my ideas off of them and express my feelings to them during this process. My husband, children, and parents, who are always so supportive. To each and every member of my family—born and chosen, friends, clients, and colleagues who encouraged, inspired, and prayed for me during this writing process.

Survey Respondents

Veronica D.

Nikke B.

Yolanda W.

Karliece A.

Cavisha W.

Aubree M.

Anonymous Participant*

G. Carter

Anonymous Participant*

M. Herron

T. Daniels

Anonymous Participant*

T. Douglas

B. Rankins

Anonymous Participant*

Toria B.

B. L.

M. Hawkins

G.O. Byrd

C. Venter

T. M.

Anonymous Participant

I appreciate each participant that took the time to thoughtfully share her thoughts, feelings, and experiences. Your heartfelt input is equally appreciated and impactful for those participants* who chose not to share their names. Thank you all!

Professional Counselors

Sasha Pinson, MS, LPC, NCC
    Licensed Professional Counselor, in San Antonio, Tx. Bachelor of Science in Psychology and Master's in Clinical Mental Health Counseling from the University of Texas in San Antonio.

Carolyn Stovall,
    B.A. in Psychology and Sociology and a minor in Women's

Studies from Bellevue College (Bellevue, Nebraska). She also has a Master's in Community Counseling from St. Mary's University (San Antonio, Texas).

Rodney Barnett, Certified Trichologist
    Dallas, Texas, USA
    Mentor and Partner

Frank Eberstadt, Author
    Corindi, New South Wales, Australia

Dr. Angela Pennington, Author
    San Antonio, Texas, USA

Vector images designed by Freepik
Celebrity photos "Balderized" by BalderaZZi.com
Social Experiment Photos – via Photoshop Pro
Author Photo by – Stephen & Staci Photography

To all of you who are living with varying degrees of hair loss and alopecia, you are the inspiration for this book. Most importantly, I want to thank God for your love; for allowing me to live my life in you, for helping me find my voice, and for allowing me to continue my ministry!

RESOURCES

American Psychiatric Association. (2022). *Diagnostic and Statistical Manual of Mental Disorders* (5th ed., text rev.). https://doi.org/10.1176/appi.books.9780890425787

Homan, K., & Hosack, L. (2019). Gratitude and the self: Amplifying the good within. *Journal of Human Behavior in the Social Environment*, *29*(7), 874–886. https://doi.org/10.1080/10911359.2019.1630345

Neal-Barnett, A., & Stadulis, R. (2006). Affective states and racial identity among African-American women with trichotillomania. *Journal of the National Medical Association*, 98(5), 753.

Shumsky, E. (2013). Discussion of Jane R. Lewis's "Hair-Pulling, Culture, and Unmourned Death." *International Journal of Psychoanalytic Self Psychology*, 8(2), 218–224. https://doi.org/10.1080/15551024.2013.768751

Snorrason, I., Belleau, E. L., & Woods, D. W. (2012). How related are hair pulling disorder (trichotillomania) and skin picking disorder? A review of evidence for comorbidity, similarities and shared etiology. *Clinical Psychology Review*, *32*(7), 618–629. https://doi.org/10.1016/j.cpr.2012.05.008.

ABOUT THE AUTHOR

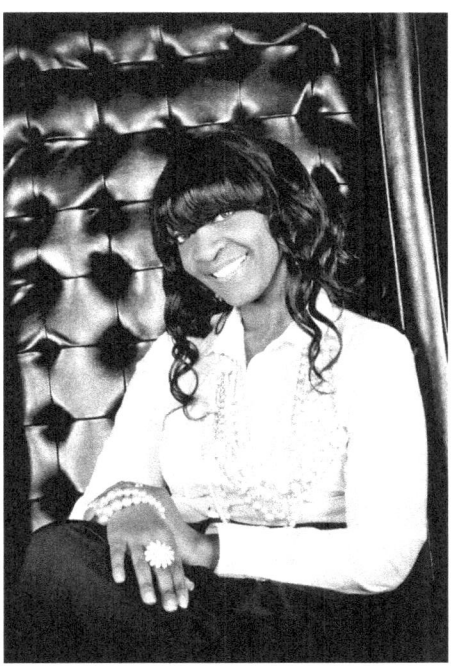

Stephanie Anderson has a true passion for the beauty industry, specializing in Hair Loss and Scalp maladies. She is the owner of Trinity Lace Wigs, The Hair Replacement Coach, the creator of the Hair Loss Pros Direct App and other endeavors and projects.

Her establishment, Trinity Lace Wigs, was created to offer exclusive hair loss replacement for women while they are battling cancer and undergoing the rigors of chemotherapy; as well as those who suffer from other forms of hair loss. She offers cranial prostheses, hair units, and wigs for women of all ages and ethnic groups. Stephanie has provided healthy hair care for over two decades. Stephanie holds certifications in Trichology, Hair Replacement, Medical Hair Loss, and Natural Health. She is a certified facilitator with the American Cancer Society's "Look Good...Feel Better" program, Better Business Bureau Torch Award Recipient, and, Who's Who in Black San Antonio Entrepreneur. She is a volunteer of the Wigs For Kids Organization, African American Leadership Institute Alum, and Certified Master Life Coach.

A licensed cosmetologist, Stephanie earned a Doctorate of Professional Cosmetology, a Master of Professional Cosmetology from the Institute of Cosmetology, and a Bachelor of Science degree in Management from the University of Phoenix. Born, raised, and educated in Oklahoma City, Stephanie now calls San Antonio home. She is the wife of Marcel Anderson, Jr., Retired Air Force, proud mother of Christian and Tristan, "GranCupcake" and "GiGi" to Beaux and Hosea.

You can connect with me on:
www.AlopeciaItsAThing.com
www.StephanieLAnderson.com
www.Facebook.com/AlopeciaItsAThing

Thanks for reading!
Please add a review on Amazon and let me know what you thought!

Amazon reviews are extremely helpful for authors, thank you for taking the time to support me and my work. Don't forget to share your review on social media with the hashtag #AlopeciaItsAThing in an effort to reach others with Alopecia and hair loss!

www.ingramcontent.com/pod-product-compliance
Lightning Source LLC
Chambersburg PA
CBHW060504130626
46553CB00002B/403